Dynamic Health,

Dismantled Obstacles

Strategy for healthy living, lifelong weight

control, and proper medication use unveiled

Dr. Oby Okoli

Library of Congress Control Number: 2013907259

Printed in the United States of America

PROLOGUE

I am delighted that you have chosen *Dynamic Health, Dismantled Obstacles.* This book adds a unique and vital dimension to healthy living. It puts medication in the proper perspective with regards to the maintenance of good health. It seeks to make us a healthier nation rather than an over-medicated nation. It broadens health consideration for various age groups for maximum benefit. It addresses important issues for long term health and has something for everyone including athletes. Several obstacles that stand in the way of good health are addressed in this book. Pivotal points on healthy living are also addressed.

As an award winning writer of health articles, I have put together information that will enable people struggling with living a healthy lifestyle to break free and live healthy. Various concerns that were raised as I collaborated with physicians and peers are addressed profitably in this book to improve health for all people. Good health for the total person was addressed from skin, weight, and organs to mental health. Even people who have chosen a healthy lifestyle will be able to broaden benefit to their health with this book. This book offers suggestions on changes that will yield benefits for life. When it comes to health, properly guided changes can yield amazing results.

Information on health can be overwhelming or even confusing. It becomes important to address specific issues on health that will offer answers to health concerns that face various people daily. This book offers a profitable balance to healthy living efforts. It brings good health within reach predictably. It makes hope of good health a reality rather than a distant dream.

DEDICATION

This book is dedicated to our Heavenly

Father, the Great and Awesome God.

I also dedicate this book to my four precious children:

Ngozi, Chidi, Chika, and Chioma

You are the best children ever!

May God bless you all.

REVIEWERS

I appreciate deeply the outstanding reviewers of this book.

I thank all of you for your diligence and sacrifice:

Joel A. Okoli, MD, MPH, FACS

Eby E. Ufondu, MD

Harvey L. Bumpers, MD, FACS

A reviewer also for National Institute of Health and several medical journals

Kyle W. Chapman, MD, FACS

Mercy N. Offor, PhD

Author of six books, including the fascinating memoir:

"REFRESHING SPRINGS: Great Legacies from a Renowned Dynasty"

It is available on amazon.com

Acknowledgement

I appreciate the valuable support from my wonderful family during the writing of this book: my husband, Dr. Joel Okoli and my children, Ngozi, Chidi, Chika, and Chioma. I also appreciate our friends/surrogate parents, Dr. & Mrs. Kyle Chapman, for their great support over the years in all our endeavors and for the support of this book. Your thoughtfulness is laudable. Thank you Dad and Mom.

I remember with gratitude to God my late parents, Mr. Daniel Nzewi and Princess Victoria Ezeokoli-Nzewi. You both were an inspiration and a blessing. You motivated all of us to achieve the highest that God has equipped us for. The legacy you both left us lives on. The godliness you instilled in us is still part of all seven of us. To my late sister Chinenye, you were amazing and unforgettable; you taught me both how to make special healthy dishes and also to garnish food with a royal touch! I want to thank also my brother, Daniel Nzewi, author, for his support and encouragement during the writing of this book, my sisters, Dr. Ify Nwabugwu and Dr. Eby Ufondu for their support, my sister, Dr. Joyce Ale, for her prayers, my brother-in-law and sister, Dozie & Grace Okonkwo, entrepreneurs, for their support, and my sister, Dr. Mercy Offor for coordinating the book efforts.

Contents

Introduction

Welcome to *Dynamic Health, Dismantled Obstacles*! This book is different from other health books. It adds a critical perspective to healthy living. It navigates you away from a vicious cycle that robs you of good health with the use of medication mask. It also addresses over 21 obstacles to healthy living. It addresses the essentials of getting healthy and staying healthy. It gives you a method of eating fruits and vegetables the right way and the easy way. It uses observations and information gathered from real people under normal and daily living circumstances. It uses surveys as well. This allows you to follow, in the book, real suggestions from real situations rather than observations from manipulated situations that are set up for a limited time or with limited people. The suggestions that are drawn from manipulated situations might not be applicable and beneficial to you.

I have made a lot of observations over the years as a healthcare professional. My years of observation of what triggers ill health and the way medications are used, prompted the writing of this book. I discuss and evaluate frequently health issues with surgeons, internists, psychiatrists, and dentists. The need to address some of the questions and health related issues that bother people also contributed to the decision to write this book. I advocate healthy living. If medications are needed, as a pharmacist, I encourage appropriate use. My pharmaceutical care suggestions detailing how to keep patients healthier, earned me a state award in the pharmaceutical care writing contest in 2000. I was also one of the pharmaceutical care award winners recognized at the American Pharmacists Association annual national conference in 2000.

The information in this book will help you live a healthier life. We are bombarded by all kinds of information today. Some of that information turns out to be very helpful and contributes positively to our lives. We also have information that we have no need for, which competes for our time and attention. It then becomes important that you invest your limited time and/or your resources in information that improves your life.

It is so important that peoples' health is steered in the right direction. People change from year to year and that is expected. However, I have seen people over the years undergo rather rapid changes in their health and appearance. These changes occurred in some cases over a matter of only two years in which I have known these people. I am not talking about people who are already very sick or diagnosed with terminal diseases. I have seen some people go rapidly, for instance, from regular size to becoming overweight or obese. I observed these changes in professional settings. I have seen some of the choices and habits that accompany these changes in health and weight. The changes seen in health and weight in these cases were very easily predictable from the observed choices and habits.

Thankfully, I have also observed two relatives go from becoming diabetics on medication to being taken off diabetic medication. This positive outcome was accomplished by adopting and adhering rigidly to a healthy lifestyle. One definitely thanks God for changes like this. In this book I will discuss some of the choices and actions that make such positive changes possible and attainable. I will also discuss the necessary steps towards accomplishing these goals.

How far are you willing to go in order to obtain and maintain good health? As far as your health is concerned, open mindedness is very profitable. Everybody is different and different people have different challenges when it comes to health and wellbeing. In this book I will look at various things that have worked for various people for so many years. You will not see any quick fix in this book. You will see, however, suggestions for simple, permanent changes that will yield positive long lasting results in your health.

Some of us want to easily see in a nut shell what it is that we need to do to improve our health. We want clear information that we can use. We obviously want something that has helped other people to achieve good results and good health. We want the efforts we put into the reading to be rewarding.

This book seeks to make available in a simple and concise fashion, knowledge that will lead to tangible changes. These tangible changes will give consistency to healthy living efforts. It is designed to eliminate guesswork as far as healthy living is concerned. Healthy living is too important to be a trial of luck kind of scenario whereby you cross your fingers and hope that whatever it is that you are told to do works for you.

If you make changes and do things differently, you ought to get a different result. If you look differently at your health and act differently and appropriately because of your health, you will be able to obtain good beneficial results. These results will profit you for the rest of your life. This book will discuss simple beneficial changes that will improve your overall health and wellbeing. My training, professional experience, interviews, and survey findings place me in a unique position to write this book.

Chapter One

Medication Mask

Your health should be polished to a shine and not dimmed with a mask. We are living in an era of excellent medical advances. Tremendous advances have been made in the provision of potent and efficacious drugs (medications). Medication options are diverse. It is awesome to know that when people are sick, they can count on solid credible medical attention. They can also count on potent medications to treat various symptoms. Our reliance on good medical attention and medications has its place. However, the availability of medications ought not to be substitutes for healthy habits and choices. Drugs are supposed to enhance health not diminish it.

I have observed for years in the pharmacy setting, as a pharmacist, the way people unknowingly use medications as health masking tapes. So many people cover themselves with "medication masking tapes" which end up diminishing their health. They are unaware of the damage being done through the use of medication masks. What are medication masking tapes? Masking tape is a tape that is used in painting. It is used to mask off various areas that should not be painted. It usually does not change the condition of the area that is masked. In other words, it covers up some areas and keeps them from receiving the attention that they will receive otherwise. Medications masks are health masking tapes. Medications as masking tapes are administered to the body when the body experiences some symptoms, in an attempt to self treat the symptoms. These symptoms are basically warning us that our bodies need some attention and that all is not well. People, unfortunately, can mask off their bodies with medications so that it is excluded from the attention that it needs and deserves. This masking of symptoms always signals trouble for future health.

Most of the people who are sick or who have been diagnosed with one medical condition or the other go through the pharmacist to complete their therapy. As a pharmacist, it is easy to see which medical conditions diagnosed in patients are preventable through lifestyle modifications. This is the case whether the sickness is treated with over the counter medications or prescription medications. Most people at one time or the other have had to use over the counter medications or prescription medications to address their ill health. Sometimes, a pattern is noticeable in patients that end up with certain medical conditions. The sickness sometimes is predictable. The good news is that prevention of a lot these illnesses or medical conditions is possible. This book will offer suggestions on how to prevent a lot of these illnesses or medical conditions.

A disturbing scenario in the use of medications as masking tape is the case of unhealthy fat consumption, for instance. Some people love steaks, hamburgers and fries. They cannot resist the enticement of juicy marbled sirloin steak cooked to perfection or

19

juicy beef hamburgers; not to mention delicious French fries. They eat these at every opportunity. They do not mind eating large sized steak such as 12 ounce marbled sirloin steak or more in one meal, (I will discuss the eating of red meat later). Usually this type of scenario will go on for some time with no noticeable concerns. However within the body, trouble will be brewing. Atherosclerotic plaque may be building up in the coronary arteries. This may reach the point that one may start to develop pain in the upper part of the abdomen or behind the sternum. This type of pain may be explained away as heart burn or even acid reflux. Consumption of readily available over the counter pain and acid reflux medications may mask the symptoms until a medical emergency interrupts the daily schedule; and one ends up in the emergency room with heart attack.

Medical evaluation and treatment follows and the famous counsel for such a scenario follows suit "Avoid saturated fat and eat healthier." Then a trip to the pharmacy is necessitated this time for one or more prescription medication(s) which is brought into the scene solely by lifestyle. This shake-up usually becomes a wake-up call for some people to remember to consider the way they eat certain things that they love. We all either know or have heard about people who have been in this situation. This is the reason why more than ever, we need to take the medication mask off so that we can live and live healthy too.

Someone told me about a parent who would take over the counter antacids on a daily basis in case he has acid reflux. He was taking the use of medication mask to a new level. He did not even wait to see if he will have acid reflux or not. He self medicated just in case he ended up needing medications. The family finally convinced him to hold off taking antacids until he had acid reflux. An even better response to a tangible symptom, be it acid reflux or other, is to note in writing what you ate or what you did differently that may have resulted in the symptom. This will enable you to isolate foods and actions that cause you problem such as acid reflux or pain. If possible, vary food or action that you think might be contributing to the symptom and note how the symptom is affected by the changes that you have made. This will help you towards establishing onset and possibly cause of symptoms. This becomes even more useful when you go to the doctor. Documenting your symptoms will allow you to give a more accurate and complete history to your doctor and facilitate your diagnosis during your doctor's visit.

In some cases your doctor will determine the reason why you are having symptoms. If the symptoms are not reflective of a serious health threat, limited use of over the counter medications may be indicated. A lot of people use over the counter medications inappropriately and for a prolonged period of time. This is a medication mask that can end up hurting you.

The body manifests symptoms to caution us that something is wrong with our bodies. It can be cautioning us that we are feeding the body something that disrupts optimal function. It can be indicating that something is deficient in our bodies and need to be replenished as in vitamin deficiency symptoms, for example, that manifest as fatigue. If we medicate the fatigue and not address the cause of the fatigue, our health problems will continue and we will get sicker. Symptoms can also indicate that something we are doing to our bodies need to be stopped. This is the case when we step on a sharp object and feel pain, or if we neglect our teeth and feel pain from them. If we medicate the pain and continue the action, we can get injured and in extreme cases get diagnosed with a serious disease. The actions of many people today seem to scream "tape it up and move on." We therefore use medications as masking tapes for health and in so doing rob ourselves of thriving health. The diseases that we invite into our lives by so doing can complicate our lives.

Obviously, certain symptoms indicate a medical emergency and others are severe enough that a prompt visit to the emergency room or the doctor is necessitated. When in doubt about how serious your symptoms are or the appropriate response to your symptoms, consult your physician to verify appropriate actions.

Take Off Medication Masks for Better Health

Medications in most cases are not the first line of action as far as interventions in health problems and health maintenance are concerned. Medications in a lot of cases are only indicated if lifestyle modifications fail to return one to good health. With your health problems you need to first answer the question, "Will lifestyle modification resolve my health problem?" Lifestyle modifications involve changes that enhance good health. If lifestyle modification can resolve your health problem, follow that pathway to regain your good health. Healthcare cost can dramatically decrease annually in the United States if people emphasize prevention rather than treatment of preventable medical conditions. Even when people are being treated with some medications, lifestyle modifications are often needed for optimal result. In other words, lifestyle modifications and healthy choices are required for better health with or without medications. It therefore makes perfect sense to use lifestyle modifications and healthy choices to prevent diseases in the first place. This is especially the case for diseases that respond to lifestyle changes.

Billions of dollars are spent each year in the United States in doctors' visits, hospital visits, and in the purchase of medications for medical conditions that are preventable. A major step towards good health is taking off medication masking tapes so that the warning symptoms by the body will receive appropriate attention that will restore normal body function and good health.

Some Drugs with Powerful Effects and Drug Cocktail

Taking medications as masking tapes includes the use of powerful drug cocktail that can make peoples' situation go from bothersome to detrimental. Unfortunately, some people attempt to obtain a quick way out in their situations. They look for a short-cut to obtaining relief. They see self treatment with medication as the answer. Some people seek to obtain "a high" from medications. This is equivalent to applying a giant masking tape of medications to real life problems. Some of these people obtain and ingest inappropriately mind altering drugs that are prescribed for somebody else. They also mix and ingest inappropriately wrong doses of powerful drugs prescribed by their doctors. The mixture of powerful drugs (cocktail) in wrong doses can lead to serious injury or even death.

Medications need to be used appropriately and only when they are indicated. Sharing prescription medications is a very bad idea. When a medication is only available by prescription, it means that its use is supposed to be initiated, monitored and supervised by a physician; advises for its use is supposed to be obtained from the dispensing pharmacist.

Indulging in prescription drugs not intended for you can impair your health or even endanger your life. Examples of such drugs include the drug group known as the benzodiazepines. Examples of drugs in this group include alprazolam and diazepam. Medications in this group are usually given for short term relief of symptoms such as anxiety, panic attack, and insomnia. These medications can be habit forming. They can cause physical and psychological dependence. This means that if you take these medications often, you can become dependent on them. If you become dependent on these medications, your body will show symptoms when you cannot have them. You might have overwhelming desire for the medications when they are not available to you. Some patients with chronic pain may have difficulty sleeping and in addition to a drug like alprazolam may also be on prescription pain medication like oxycodone and acetaminophen. The premise is that these medications will be taken appropriately as instructed.

Combining these medications in a cocktail is like opting for injury predictably and rapidly. Some people enjoy the state of mind the drug puts them in when mixed in a cocktail. These people do not realize that the state of mind it puts them in can be a major step on the path of injury from the combined drug effects. Unfortunately, it is like driving one's car off the cliff in order to get the thrill similar to that from a roller coaster ride. No one would drive a car off the cliff and get injured just to obtain a transient feeling and yet people fail to understand that this scenario is the same as consuming a drug cocktail with powerful drugs. It is a situation where lack of understanding and misconception of a thrill can cause people some injury and traumatize their loved ones and others who care about them.

Suggestions for Powerful Drugs and Drug Cocktail

If you are in a situation or mental state where you need to block out consciousness to get you through a day or through a phase in your life, the last thing you need is a powerful mind altering drug cocktail. There is a big difference between blocking your mind out and causing yourself harm. The drug cocktail cannot distinguish between mind block and injury. Taking them in that way can do both, leaving you with no net benefit. If you escape injury after consuming a cocktail of powerful drugs at any time, remember one thing. The fact that you escaped injury with the ingestion of drug cocktail of powerful drugs is an exception rather than an expected outcome in your situation. What drugs in a cocktail have to offer you, unfortunately, include threat to your life.

If getting through your day is a big challenge for you, the thing that will help you and give you a beneficial outcome and long lasting benefit is a miracle of restoration. Seek help through sound, caring counseling. Seek prayers as well. So many people have been able to get back on the right tract and so can you. There was a man whose life was very far from being normal. Anyone who can dress themselves and carry out any life function is in a better situation than this man was. He was extremely troubled. His life was returned to normal through a miracle of restoration by Jesus. His story was recorded in Mark 5:1-20.

Choose and walk in the direction of health. Do not allow yourself to be in the path of ultimate demise. Continue to get help. Avoid the temptation to resort to a quick fix. Choose to let go the use of medication masking tape. Your situation may be impossible right now but remember that in the big picture of your life this might be just a tough page and not the whole book of your life. Be hopeful and stay positive. Surround yourself with love, support, and help.

Inappropriate Dependence on Medications

Medications have their place in peoples' health. If used appropriately, they can be beneficial. They can help an asthmatic patient breath better, for instance. When medications are used outside of their appropriate indications, they can be a hindrance to health and in some cases cause harm. Several patients have brought to my attention the fact that the doctor whom they saw did not prescribe any medication to them. I want our patients to get the medications that they need, however, medications are not indicated sometimes when someone goes to see a doctor.

Some children seem to be full of energy and they engage in restless activities. Keeping up with these children can be quite a challenge from day to day. At some point, they get placed on medications.

Suggestions for Inappropriate Dependence on Medications

When it comes to symptoms in a lot of cases, it is vital to maintain the right order; first lifestyle modifications and second medications. It is not the other way around. I encourage lifestyle modification whenever it is appropriate. There are some exceptions to this situation such as a confirmed infection.

Children who participate significantly in sports and activities are more easily focused and purposeful. Sports and other activities can give children a sense of accomplishment. First allow your child to participate in sports and other activities such as the playing of musical instruments, dancing, and creative drawing. Be sure to get them into major physical activities daily. They will be naturally exhausted and would have much less energy for destructive activities. They might even discover a talent that they have in the process. This approach towards raising energetic children will reduce the number of children who are on daily medications.

Some medications have major side effects which can diminish overall health over time. Some medications are used only on one basis. This basis is that the benefits of using such medications outweigh the risk of suffering with the symptom or disease state for which the medications are prescribed. Medications are useful but they should always be used when appropriate and not as the first line of action.

Seven Do's and Don'ts Regarding Taking Medications

Seven Do's Regarding Taking Medications

(1) Do store medications away from heat, direct light, moisture, and children.

(2) Do eat first, always, before taking any nonsteroidal anti-inflammatory drug (NSAID) such as aspirin, ibuprofen, and naproxen. This will help you to avoid damage to your stomach lining, avoid ulcer, and consequently avoid bleeding.

(3) Do take all medications as directed by your prescriber.

(4) Do add healthy diet and exercise to your medication intake for your medical conditions such as high cholesterol, high blood pressure, diabetes, obesity, and other conditions.

(5) Do associate the intake of your medication with time or activity to enable you remember to take your medication. For example, if your medication is three times a day, take it around breakfast, lunch, and dinner. If empty stomach is needed, then take it one hour before you eat or two hours after you eat. If it is once a day medication, take it around breakfast or around dinner depending on the type of medication. If it is once a week medication, take it on a

meeting day such as before a Wednesday meeting. If it is once a month medication, take it on the first day of the month or on the last day of the month.

(6) Do take whole any medication that has controlled release (CR), extended release [(ER), XR and XL], or sustained release (SR) indication. Do not break or crush them as that will disrupt their action. Some of them have 'shells' and because of that, they are eliminated from your body looking like they did when you took them.

(7) Do review thoroughly the information on your medication that is given to you with it. Do this for every medication that you receive until you become familiar with the medication.

Seven Don'ts Regarding Taking Medications

(1) Do not ignore muscle aches and muscle weakness that start for no reason after you start certain medications. The medications that can cause muscle aches and weakness include the medication group known as the statins used to treat high cholesterol. An example of such a medication is simvastatin. The muscle aches or weakness happens only in some cases. If this type of medication side effect occurs, it is indicating muscle damage risk. You need to discontinue the medication and promptly report the problem to your physician. Do not "tough it out."

(2) Do not treat dry persistent cough with over the counter medications if it started as a result of taking certain medications. Medications that cause dry cough include the Angiotensin Converting Enzyme (ACE) Inhibitors used to treat high blood pressure. An example of ACE inhibitor is lisinopril. The generic versions of these medications usually end in –pril. Let the doctor know if you get bothersome dry cough on these medications and the doctor will switch you to another medication.

(3) Do not take acetaminophen for a long period of time beyond seven days unless directed to do otherwise by your physician. Limit amount and limit duration of acetaminophen therapy. This is because taking large amounts of acetaminophen over a short period of time could damage the liver and cause liver failure. Do not take acetaminophen from more than one source at the same time. For example, do not take acetaminophen over the counter and oxycodone with acetaminophen or hydrocodon with acetaminophen. This could result in your taking large amount of acetaminophen over a short period of time which could damage your liver.

(4) Do not discontinue prescribed maintenance or daily medications on your own without consulting your physician. Your physician will wean you off of your medications safely when you no longer need them.

(5) Do not ignore any bothersome symptoms or side effects that start after you start taking your medications. This includes itching, rash, hives, fever, or shortness of breath. Stop the medication and let your doctor know. This can occur with certain medications to which you are allergic.

(6) Do not take expired medications. Be aware of the expiration dates of your medications.

(7) Do not stop your antibiotics before you are supposed to unless advised to do so by your physician. Always take your antibiotics until all of them are finished even if you feel better after a couple of days of therapy. If you discontinue the antibiotics prematurely, the bacteria being treated (that are still remaining) will develop resistance to the antibiotics that you were taking. The next time that antibiotic is prescribed for you or for somebody else, it will be ineffective. This will decrease the number of effective antibiotics available to people. It is a major medical concern. Take antibiotics with plenty of water unless directed otherwise. This will facilitate the elimination of the antibiotics.

Caution Concerning Medications

Symptoms can be relieved or controlled by products that range from simple saline nasal sprays to serious chemical substances. Medications manufactured using serious chemical substances can facilitate healing or control of medical conditions when used appropriately. When used inappropriately, they can be dangerous or harmful. This is why there are guidelines, counsel, and precautions for their use. When medications are indicated, take the right amount, in the right way always.

Brand Versus Generic Medications: Which Should I Buy?

Difference between Brand Name Medications and Generic Medications

As a pharmacist, I get a lot of questions from patients concerning brand and generic medications. Patients want to know if they should buy the brand or the generic medication. In some cases, the brand name medication is two to three times the price of the generic. Some people believe that the brand name medication must be doing more than the generic medication or it will not be much more expensive. This is why some patients look at the pharmacist sometimes during medication counseling as if to say, "Am I missing something?" This is in response to being told that they can buy the brand name medication or the generic. Usually brand name medications undergo expensive clinical trials to establish safety and efficacy before they are approved and marketed. This contributes immensely to the high price of brand name medications. The generic medications do not undergo clinical trials so they are much cheaper to produce.

Medications contain two types of ingredients. The two types of ingredients are the active ingredients and the excipients. The excipients are the inactive ingredient component of the medication. For any drug to qualify as a generic drug, it must contain the same active ingredient as the brand name medication. The key difference between the brand name and the generic medications that are marketed is the excipients contained in the medications. The brand and the generic medications therefore contain the same active ingredient. They may contain different inactive ingredients.

The brand and generic medications are therefore equally effective because of the active ingredient. You can choose to buy the brand or the generic medication and that is alright. If price is a concern for you, then buy the cheaper one which is usually the generic medication. The only time that the one you choose is important is if you are bothered by any of the inactive ingredients. Some people may have some discomfort or adverse reaction to some of the excipients in certain medications. This situation is very rare. If this happens to you while taking a generic medication, you can switch to the brand name medication. If you have a reason, otherwise to believe that you fare better with the brand name medications, go ahead and buy brand name medications.

How about Pain Medications?

Special consideration of pain medications is worthwhile. Generic pain medications are widely dispensed and they have been very effective for the control of pain for a lot of people. Some people, however, say that generic pain medications do not effectively control their pain. If you believe that the brand name option works better for your pain, especially where pain control can be jeopardized, you can buy the brand name pain medications. Pain control is very important, however, I will strongly discourage overuse of pain medications. Some people even create their own dose by doubling the recommended dose. This should be avoided at all cost. A better solution, than the overuse of pain medications to control pain, is to work with your physician until pain control is achieved. There are a lot of options to choose from.

Preventing Illness and Seven Germ Carriers People May Overlook

Preventing Illness with Germicides and Germicide Wipes

People encounter germs everyday that in some cases lead to illness. In some situations the germs spread to healthy people from those who are already sick. Hand washing with soap when available especially after using the bathroom is very effective in reducing infection. However, when unavailable, germicides and germicide wipes which are currently available in most public places are very helpful in decreasing germs that can make people sick. This is especially true if these germicides are used effectively and at appropriate times. When it comes to health, prevention of a disease is much better than the pursuit of a cure.

Unfortunately, some people overlook certain sources of germs and therefore make themselves vulnerable to these germs by so doing. Having a phobia for germs is not necessary. However, it is good to be aware of various germ carriers in order to effectively avoid the sickness caused through the exposure to these germs. It is not by accident that young children who go to daycare become sick. Some of these children get sick rather frequently, and others some of the time. Young children share a lot of things. They are unable to take the precautions that are necessary to avoid germs that can make them sick. In some cases, these young children pass the sickness to the adults in their homes who can in turn pass it to other adults.

As part of helpful precaution, adults can ensure that children wash their hands thoroughly with soap and water before leaving the daycare. The clothes worn to the daycare at the end of each day should also be washed with disinfectants.

Seven Germ Carriers People May Overlook

(1) Public nursery toys shared by children

(2) Public pens and writing surfaces

(3) Public bathroom sink or vanity countertop

(4) Public computer keyboards

(5) Money; coins and currencies

(6) Public door knobs

(7) Hands (of persons who happen to be sick) during handshake

Taking advantage of the availability of germicides is a good step towards keeping healthy. People strive to keep their hands clean, but sick people might not be able to avoid completely contact between their hands and the germs that have made them sick. Being aware of this will encourage people to take necessary precautions to remain healthy.

Seven Increases that You Need to Avoid

Expansion or increase can be a very good thing. It could be a sign of progress. There are areas, however, where increased frequency or increase in size or amount is not a good thing. These represent increases that you do not need.

Increases in the area of health that you need to avoid are;

(1) Increase in junk food consumption

(2) Increase in your waistline

(3) Ongoing increase in your weight

(4) Increase in poor health choices

(5) Increase in symptoms due to neglect of health

(6) Increase in catastrophic habits that adversely affect your health

(7) Increase in your medication collection, especially for those disease states that are preventable

Action Summary # 1

Avoid taking medications as the first step when you have a symptom. We have seen that medication is not the first line of action in health situations. Try to establish wherever possible why the symptom started and when the symptom started. This will enable the right action to be taken at the right time; which will help in restoring good health. It will also ensure that health warning signs and symptoms are not covered up or masked with medications; as this would cause health to deteriorate. Furthermore it will help you to give a better history of your situation to your doctor.

Obtain medical advice when you have symptoms. If the symptoms are not indications of a serious health threat, a limited use of over the counter medication may be indicated. A lot of people use over the counter medications inappropriately and for a prolonged period of time. Avoid using over the counter medications in this way because if used inappropriately they could end up doing more harm than good.

Protect your health by using medications only when it is indicated and only how it is indicated. Do not take medications if lifestyle modifications will make the medication unnecessary. Lifestyle modification alone can help to resolve a lot of medical conditions.

Whether you buy the brand or the generic medication, you are obtaining the required active ingredient in that medication. If you are not bothered in some way by either one, buy whichever is convenient for you.

Wash hands when needed. Use germicides and germicide wipes to protect your health. There are several germ carriers that some people may overlook. Seven of such germ carriers are listed in this chapter. They include toys that children share in public nurseries. They also include public computer key boards.

Increase can be a good thing but avoid increase in unprofitable areas such as weight, waistline, junk food consumption, and poor health choices. Avoid also increase in symptoms due to the neglect of your health.

If you follow the suggestions in this book, a lot of symptoms that indicate ill health can be avoided and you will be healthier.

Chapter Two

Health Overview

Good health is priceless. No effort or sacrifice made towards it is too much. There are certain steps we must take and others we must avoid to obtain it. This book will help you prepare yourself to obtain good health.

It is interesting to see how on a daily basis we can move our lives in directions that over time prove to be very rewarding. However, there are certain steps that can be taken that over time hinder our progress in many ways. We do this sometimes unconsciously. The driving force behind the direction towards which we move our lives is simply choice. Choice when appropriate can be wonderful and when inappropriate becomes a hindrance. Some people wonder why we should have the freedom of choice since we end up making so many wrong choices that end up hurting us. Choice is supposed to be a good thing. A choice that ends up hurting us is definitely not a good thing. That makes it necessary to qualify choice. Guarded appropriate choice is a good thing. When a choice is guarded it means that the choice has been screened for negative effects. When a choice is appropriate, it means that it is expected to yield good outcome. Our choices ought to meet these two criteria always and health choices are no different.

Every day we wake up we are faced with a lot of health choices whether we realize and acknowledge them or not. Every day we go to bed we have made a lot of health choices whether we noticed them or not. Every week we go through we have moved ourselves forwards or backwards in terms of our health. Every New Year, we are faced with opportunities of all kinds of new choices. At the end of every year we have made several choices that have either disturbed or refreshed our health.

A lot of people ask me questions about healthy living. Some people run their food choices by me and ask for my advice. Others admit to cravings for foods and snacks which they know are unhealthy and ask for my suggestion. I have also had some of the people discuss their exercise choices with me. I have even had some people change what they eat since they started being around me and these people will inform me of the changes they have made in what they eat. For some reason, I seem to attract healthy lifestyle discussions. I am absolutely passionate about healthy living. It gives me joy to help anyone in any way to live healthier. There is, however, a limit to what I can say to people about health in answer to their questions or while counseling people as a health care professional. One of the reasons for writing this book is to help people implement steps to good health in a simple, concise, and adoptable style.

A Bridge for the Divide

Bridges play crucial roles in everyday life. They connect you to your destinations. They allow you to go from where you are to where you need to be. A bridge is important also when it comes to a healthy lifestyle and good health. There are two critical components of your bridge to good health. Combining and utilizing these two components will allow you to go from having knowledge alone to the implementation of knowledge and achieving good health. Ignoring or neglecting these two components will jeopardize your chances of achieving and maintaining a healthy lifestyle and good health.

These two critical components of the bridge to good health are:

Determination and
Commitment

These two principles enabled Daniel (*Belteshazzar*) and his friends, Hananiah (*Shadrach*), Mishael (*Meshach*), and Azariah (*Abednego*) to win the very first health contest which was recorded in the Bible. The story is found in the Book of Daniel Chapter one in the Bible.

Daniel's 10 Days a Vegetarian Challenge (The First Clinical Trial Ever)

The importance of healthy eating is not a new concept. Daniel was aware of this concept and applied it in a contest. This very contest had to do with health and appearance. He used tools that cannot fail.

First, Daniel had a determination; he "made up his mind." He determined not to defile himself with certain foods and drinks. He proposed a healthy eating and a healthy look challenge or contest. Foods and looks are always related. "Test us for ten days," he said; "give us vegetables to eat and water to drink. Then compare us with the young men who are eating the food of the royal court, and base your decision on how we look." Daniel 1:12-13 (Good News Bible, GNB). Daniel and his three friends, therefore, became participants in a health contest. *This is the first ever reported clinical trial in the history of mankind.*

Secondly, Daniel committed to his determination. In this particular challenge, result was everything. A lot of decisions depended on the outcome of this challenge. At the end of the 10 days the results were in. The verdict was that Daniel and his friends won the health contest because "they looked healthier and stronger than all those who had been eating the royal food." Daniel 1:15, (GNB). He and his friends incorporated this healthy eating into their daily lives because they continued the healthy eating for three years. At the end of three years they were placed in very responsible positions.

When it comes to healthy living, persistence makes you a winner. Like Daniel, we have today the option of eating a variety of foods and drinking a variety of beverages some of which are in fact toxic to our bodies in the long run. I will discuss how you too can win life's health contest, in spite of some obstacles.

Health Considerations

The most important thing you can do about your health and weight is to build a bridge for the divide that keeps you from good health and weight. Make a determination and commit to what needs to be done. Doing what needs to be done gets you where you need to be. Healthy thinking will result in consistent healthy actions and consistent healthy actions will result in a healthy body. You need to think about what your body needs for you to be healthy. Make available to your body what it needs to be healthy, move your body in a way to keep it healthy and enjoy good health and good weight as a result.

Thinking about the Needs of Your Body

We have all heard that it is very important to eat right, exercise, and live a healthy lifestyle. In spite of this widespread information on the need to be healthy, a lot of people are still unable to pay adequate attention to their health. We can all come up with legitimate reasons why we cannot go from hearing what is good for our health to doing what is good for our health. We can also do what is good for our health as a project and not as a lifestyle. Health projects often get abandoned and end up unsuccessful long term. This can leave us discouraged. It can also make us give up on healthy efforts.

It is very easy to go about life doing whatever is convenient at any point in time. For instance, it might be convenient to go about our day eating whatever we are accustomed to eating or eating whatever we like as much as we want. It is also possible to end our day tired with little profitable movement or exercise and possibly end up with insufficient rest at night. We could live like this for sometime without even noticing anything wrong with our bodies. Overtime however, our bodies develop symptoms that will send us to the doctor and maybe to the hospital in addition.

When it comes to cars, we have the right mindset and think the right thoughts towards our cars. We learn what our cars need and do just that to ensure optimal functioning of our cars. A lot of us even go the extra mile to give our cars the treatment that we can be proud of.

Our bodies just like cars need good maintenance. We put the right fuel in the car to enable it run optimally. We do not just take our cars to any convenient service station when it requires maintenance. For maintenance, we all take our cars to the right service station wherever that is located. We basically give our cars all that they need to perform very well. Unfortunately sometimes, we give our bodies the wrong 'fuel,' neglect its maintenance, and make minimal investment towards maintaining healthy bodies. Our bodies as a result malfunction. When our bodies malfunction, depending on the extent of damage and depending on what is damaged in our bodies, we become unhealthy. Sometimes the performance of our daily functions could be adversely affected if our bodies malfunction.

45

What the car mechanics tell you about your car is also true of the body. Car mechanics tell you that if you maintain your car promptly and appropriately, it will save you expensive repairs on the long run. Similarly, if you maintain your body appropriately and pay attention to your health, it will save you expensive and sometimes painful trips to the hospital and pharmacy. It could even save your life. Remember that your daily actions have health outcomes that can be good or bad. As far as good health is concerned think long term. For instance, if you continue with your current habits think of how your health will be affected five or ten years from now. Channel your efforts to healthy actions that will suit your lifestyle and become a part of you. Consistent healthy actions are critical to good health and energy.

Healthy lifestyle and its results need not be seen as unattainable. When it comes to a healthy lifestyle and good health, you need to take a bold step from being a cheer leader to becoming the main player. Position yourself for success and become a winner in this area of life.

Unfortunately, age gets blamed for some of the wrong things that happen as a result of poor choices. You will often hear people say, "Oh! I am not as active now that I am older, as I was in my younger years." How old is older exactly? I once heard about a lady who was in her seventies and was still as active as ever. A closer attention to this situation revealed that there was no accident about this situation. This lady had chosen good health and energy by the way she thought, ate, and exercised her body. What we put in is reflected in what we manifest when it comes to our health, weight, and fitness.

Gene is often blamed for various conditions that result in poor health. Always remember that you may have a risk factor through your gene but having a risk factor does not guarantee the manifestation of a health condition or disease. The presence of a risk factor (or several risk factors) alone is not all that it takes to become unhealthy. A risk factor, in some cases, is a forewarning to proactively avoid a particular health condition by taking no chances with prevention. You cannot help what you cannot change but you ought to change what you can help. Again, you may be unable to change the gene, but you can determine to change the microenvironment! Do not defeat yourself by giving up on what you can change for you to be healthy.

Reality

People come in various shapes and sizes, having various likes, dislikes, as well as, various habits, and tendencies. Natural uncontrolled size, desires, habits, and tendencies can result in a lot of trouble and endanger one's health. Uncontrolled size leads to sickness and reduced energy. Uncontrolled desire leads to addiction, sickness, and even death, while uncontrolled habits jeopardize health in various ways. As far as your health is concerned, you cannot desire and enjoy the same things, maintain the same habits, and hope to obtain a different look and a successful health outcome. If you are not getting the needed result in your health or weight, then change is indicated.

Some Issues Surrounding Weight

Health awareness efforts are now widespread. The need for active roles by people towards healthier lives is clear. There is a lot of concern today about weight. Two extreme groups of people have emerged as far as weight situations are concerned.

The first group of people has become so concerned about weight that they are willing to do things that are inappropriate and potentially harmful to achieve their ideal weight or even stay thin.

Using Unhealthy Measures to Lose Weight and Stay Thin

Inappropriate measures used to lose weight and stay thin include; starvation, habits of binge and purge, and the use of laxatives to get rid of the foods that have been eaten. These methods of weight control are unhealthy and can lead to ill health.

Health problems that can arise from unhealthy weight loss measures include;

    (1) Dehydration
    (2) Irregular heath beat
    (3) Low blood pressure
    (4) Dry skin
    (5) Abdominal pain

(6) Constipation

(7) Amenorrhea

(8) Being cold frequently

(9) Damage of teeth and gums from repeated eating and
    purging

The second group is so concerned about not being the right weight, in spite of some efforts, that they have given up altogether and have become overweight or obese. Obesity results in ill health as well.

Excess Weight Issues and Disease States

Why Should You Be Concerned with Being Overweight or Obese?

Being overweight or obese has consequences that go beyond cosmetic considerations. If cosmetic considerations and ability to perform daily functions are the only concerns with being overweight or obese, I would not worry about it as much. This is because I have seen a lot of big and beautiful people who perform their daily functions like they are supposed to. We all know some people who are big and beautiful. However, my concern with anyone being overweight or obese pertains to health issues. Extra weight slowing you down is only one of the problems of being overweight or obese.

Some medical conditions and disease states can be precipitated by excess weight and fat. Also some medical conditions and disease states can be exacerbated by excess weight and fat. These disease states diminish the quality of life and the lifespan.

Some Disease States from Excess Weight

Disease states that can be precipitated or exacerbated by excess weight include:

(1) Type II diabetes or Adult Onset diabetes

(2) Coronary artery disease (CAD)

(3) High blood pressure (HBP)

(4) High cholesterol (HC)

(5) Osteoarthritis (OA)

Type II Diabetes or Adult-Onset Diabetes or Non-Insulin Dependent Diabetes

The carbohydrates that we eat are processed in different ways by the body. They can be digested and converted into blood glucose. They can also remain undigested by the human body and are known as fiber. Glucose is used to provide the energy that the body needs. Problems result in the body when blood glucose levels are too low (hypoglycemia). Symptoms are manifested in the body because of these problems. There is also a problem in the body when the blood glucose levels are too high (hyperglycemia). Symptoms are also manifested due to high blood glucose levels.

Symptoms of hyperglycemia include:

(1) Polyuria (Frequent or excessive urination)

(2) Polydipsia (Frequent or excessive thirst)

(3) Headache

(4) Fatigue

(5) Vision problem (Blurry vision)

(6) Shortness of breath (Eventually if not corrected)

(7) Confusion (Eventually if not corrected)

Symptoms of hypoglycemia include:

(1) Hunger

(2) Headache

(3) Sweating

(4) Anxiety

(5) Shaking

(6) Blurred vision (Eventually if not treated)

(7) Slurred speech or problem when trying to speak (Eventually if not treated)

(8) Confusion (Eventually if not treated)

The human body, however, has mechanisms in place that help it to control blood glucose. There are two situations that can make blood glucose levels to increase and remain high. One of the situations is when the body is unable to make sufficient insulin. The other situation is when the body is not sensitive to available insulin. When blood glucose level increases and remains high, diabetes results.

 A lot of Americans suffer from Type II or Adult Onset diabetes. Weight tremendously influences the development of Type II diabetes. Furthermore, weight influences the diabetic medication therapy. The dose and the quantity of anti-diabetic medications included in the medication plan are affected by weight. Diabetes can be influenced by what people eat.

Type II diabetes has negative consequences. The negative consequences that can result due to Type II diabetes include:

> (1) Vision problems or even blindness
> (2) Kidney failure (major cause of kidney failure in the US)
> (3) Loss of limbs (through amputation) eventually if diabetes is not adequately controlled
> (4) Increased bacterial infection in mouth and skin
> (5) Increased fungal infection in mouth and skin
> (6) Increased risk of heart attack
> (7) Increased risk of stroke

Dramatic decrease in weight or the return to one's ideal weight can minimize Type II diabetes or enhance the resolution of Type II diabetes in people. Some people have actually been taken off all their anti-diabetic medications due to adherence to lifestyle changes. Uncontrolled diabetes can complicate life in so many ways.

Coronary Artery Disease (CAD)

Coronary arteries feed the heart. They supply the heart with oxygen as well as nutrients. Plaques, which are filled with cholesterol, can build up in the arteries thereby narrowing and hardening the arteries and resulting in CAD. Plaques consist not only of cholesterol, but also of fat and other substances in the blood. CAD therefore can be precipitated by a lot of body fat. The usual cause of CAD is the atherosclerotic obstruction of the vessels which can eventually lead to heart attack. Heart attack is also called myocardial infarction. Unfortunately, it is possible to have atherosclerosis with no signs or symptoms and sometimes heart attack is the first manifestation. CAD in a lot of cases results in congestive heart failure (CHF).

High Blood Pressure (HBP)

High blood pressure or hypertension (HBP) results when blood pressure cannot be controlled. It causes the heart to work harder than usual. HBP is the primary risk factor for heart disease which includes heart failure. HBP is also a risk factor for stroke.

Some cases of HBP occur as a result of the thickening of arterial vessel wall, a condition known as arteriosclerosis.

Atherosclerosis is a type of arteriosclerosis in which vessel walls thicken and harden due to fat deposits. Narrowing of vessels adversely affects blood flow and increase blood pressure and sustained increase in blood pressure can result in a heart attack.

High Cholesterol (HC)

High cholesterol or hypercholesterolemia (HC) is a problem as well. It is the presence in the blood of high levels of cholesterol. High density lipoprotein (HDL) also known as good cholesterol has protective effects on the body. Low density lipoprotein (LDL) also known as bad cholesterol, on the other hand, has damaging effects on blood vessels. Diets high in cholesterol can result in elevated levels of cholesterol in the blood. Obesity is a risk factor for HC.

Changes in cholesterol and phospholipids metabolism (or breakdown) play a role in arteriosclerosis. So HBP, HC, and CAD are related and I call them the "terrible trio." If you are diagnosed with HBP, watch out for the other two members of the "terrible trio," (that is HC and CAD).

Osteoarthritis (OA)

Osteoarthritis is a disease in which there is degeneration of the cartilage and the underlying bone. Pain occurs in weight bearing joints, as well as joint stiffness with osteoarthritis over time. Obesity is considered a risk factor for developing osteoarthritis of the knee.

The five disease states discussed above have been linked to excess weight or fat. So if you are obese, you have increased chance of having HBP, HC, CAD, and OA in addition to obesity.

Addressing Weight

Addressing weight by itself and not as an integral part of a healthy lifestyle is a lopsided perspective, which is likely to fall short. This is why some people focus on weight quick fixes or adopt unprofitable weight and diet measures and end up with failure. We need to emphasize a healthy lifestyle and good healthy weight is part of the benefit of adhering to a healthy lifestyle. There needs to be a major shift from weight frenzy rollercoaster to the adoption of a healthy lifestyle. Everyone will profit from this.

This maintenance of a healthy weight is not the same thing as a demand that you look like someone else or any model. It is a case by case situation where the idea is to evaluate, implement, and maintain a healthy lifestyle and weight and consequently become a healthier you.

Some people have the motto of "eat whatever you want and lose weight." Weight loss alone is not enough for good health. You can eat food that can increase your cholesterol, clog your arteries and diminish your health and wellbeing and you could be at risk of a heart attack and stroke in spite of reduced weight. A healthy lifestyle is a powerful tool for improved health and good energy. Wellbeing is really being in good health and being happy.

In spite of the knowledge that we need to eat the right food, maintain the right weight, and take good care of ourselves, millions of Americans and people worldwide are overweight and obese. Everyone knows someone who is overweight and everyone knows somebody who is obese. Some people have family members, or friends, or neighbors, or co-workers who are either overweight or obese. Some people have actually surrounded themselves, knowingly or unknowingly, with lifestyles and habits that consistently increase their weight and after sometime they seem trapped in these lifestyles and habits and helplessly go along with it. This is not about acquiring a particular look. It is about maintaining a healthy body. It is important to remember that even though no one owes another person a particular size or look, the human body does not fare very well with excess weight or fat.

While on vacation in Orlando Florida in August of 2010, I casually surveyed 500 people and about one out of four people in my survey was obese. This is in spite of my excluding borderline obese people. I surveyed people at two major attractions. If I included borderline obese people, it would have been one out of three people that are obese. If I combined obese and overweight people and compared them to people with healthy weight, the ratio of obese and overweight people to people with healthy weight will be worse than one out of three people.

Is Eating Pattern Due to Cost or Choice?

One could argue that healthy food could be expensive. One could also say that people gain weight because they cannot afford healthy food. The question then is, "Are people overweight always because of the higher cost of healthy food; or are some people overweight because of their eating habits?" My vacation in the summer of 2011 made me wonder whether cost is really the biggest reason why people eat unhealthy.

At a cruise with my family in the summer of 2011, the ship provided unlimited healthy foods. There were fresh fruits, vegetables, and various foods for breakfast and lunch. For dinner you had a choice of a healthy dinner in the restaurant. In spite of this generous provision of healthy food choices, some people chose pastries. They served themselves, from the buffet, several servings of pastries. Clearly, this indicated an unhealthy habit. This is because the buffet items were available to everybody in the ship. This is at no additional cost.

To my surprise, the pizza bar was extremely popular even at night. The pizza that a lot of the people were eating had regular crust. Eating pizza, often, during the day or even once every day is not recommended among daily healthy foods. High glycemic index foods cause a spike in blood glucose when eaten. I will briefly discuss the concept of glycemic index later. A habit of eating a generous amount of high glycemic index foods such as pizza is not good for you. It is even worse if you eat the high glycemic index food as a late night meal or snack.

The expectation was that people on the vacation will gain weight. In the ship for the period of seven days, the expected weight gain was an average of eight pounds. I ate until my husband laughed at me daily. As a result of my food choices, however, I gained only three and one-half pounds at the end of the seven-day trip. Upon returning home, I rapidly lost this extra weight in a few days without even planning for any weight loss.

Change or fluctuations in a person's weight, from time to time, is a fact of life. Someone on vacation as seen above might gain weight. Someone might gain weight around Christmas. Extreme stress can cause someone to experience weight loss. Extremely busy schedule can also cause somebody to lose weight. Consistent weight gain over time, however, is an issue that needs careful attention.

There is concern if you gain weight consistently over time after you have adopted and adhered to a healthy lifestyle. Also there is concern if you are eating the right portion of the right food and still gaining weight. This type of unexpected weight gain might be due to an underlying and undiagnosed medical condition that needs prompt medical attention.

Seven Wrong Reasons to Eat: Contributors to F.L.A.B

Flab can be defined as undesirable body fat. F.L.A.B., however, stands in my opinion for the following;

F: Food

L: Lover's

A: Augmentation (Enlargement)

B: Battle

Seven wrong reasons to eat that contribute to F.L.A.B. include the following;

(1) Using food as an antidepressant by eating when depressed or discouraged
(2) Using food to combat boredom by eating when bored
(3) Eating food for companionship when lonely
(4) Eating food for enjoyment to feel happy
(5) Eating food for fun to feel good
(6) Eating food when stressed to combat stress
(7) Eating food for relaxation

Win Against F.L.A.B

In the daily struggle with F.L.A.B, become a winner. If you eat for the above reasons, consider replacing food with beneficial activities. When you are missing a companion, connect with other people in a way that is most convenient for you.

Avoid eating when you are not hungry. Avoid staying where you have easy access to food. Consider the end result of eating unnecessarily. When you eat inappropriately, you are likely to gain weight and this can result in ill health.

False hopes concerning weight loss include:

(a) Having a quick weight loss diet that end up being temporal and regaining weight lost at the end of dieting.

(b) Having an emotional plan for weight loss such as desiring to fit into certain clothes or look like certain people rather than making permanent lifestyle changes.

(c) Having a surgical procedure to enhance weight loss without accounting for a means of maintaining the weight after the surgery.

Three Keys to Healthy Weight Maintenance:

The ability to maintain a healthy weight does not happen by accident. There are healthy actions that result in a healthy weight as a consequence.

The three keys to healthy weight maintenance include;

(1) A plan which involves lifestyle modifications that will help you to achieve as well as maintain a healthy weight

(2) Thinking in a realistic and profitable way about your health as it relates to your weight

60

(3) Lifestyle of adhering to healthy choices, keeping active, and eating the right foods

I. A Plan Which Involves Lifestyle Modifications that Will Help You to Achieve as well as Maintain a Healthy Weight

Develop a healthy living plan. This plan should involve the daily healthy foods that you should eat, the type of physical daily movement or exercise you need to adopt and good rest. I will look at healthy eating recommendations and also exercises that you can plan from in later chapters. Involve an accountability partner. This partner is the person who will hold you accountable for adhering to a healthy lifestyle that will result in weight loss and weight maintenance.

The plan should also involve, at least in the beginning, a journal entry. The journal entry should have all the things that you plan to eat and the exercises you plan to do daily and how consistently you are doing them. It should also have your weight measurements as you go along each week. At the end of each week, adjust your plan if weight loss is not favored and maintain your plan if weight loss is favored. Once your plan starts to yield desired weight outcome, maintain the plan that consistently favor weight loss until you are within your ideal weight range. The journal will help you to keep focused on the right actions until you get used to them and until they become part of your daily life. A plan that is good for you should easily fit into your lifestyle so that you will be able to follow it without difficulty daily.

To enhance your success, recognize and identify everything that contribute to your weight gain. Devise a strategy to combat each contributor to weight gain and each excuse you have that favor weight gain. Make weight friendly adjustments and keep to them.

Contributors to Weight Gain

An example of a contributor to weight gain is a habit of eating daily a type of snack that gets converted rapidly into blood glucose. Remove this obstacle to healthy weight by eating healthier 100% natural snacks.

Another example of a contributor to weight gain is dinner time. Some people get back from work late most days of the week. Consequently, they eat dinner between 9:00 and 11:00pm or even later on most days of the week. It has been extremely difficult for some people to lose weight while eating dinner very late at night. I know some people who found it impossible to lose weight in spite of trying for a long time until dinner time adjustment was made. To overcome this obstacle to a healthy weight, take your dinner to work if you are working late and eat it by 7:00pm or as early as you can. If you are hungry later, snack on a high fiber vegetable such as carrots and broccoli. If you have unresolved diabetes, you would need to be cautious about your night time blood glucose level. It would be best to work with your physician concerning the maintenance of appropriate night time blood glucose levels. If you need to get it up at night, you can have an apple.

A third contributor to weight gain is mindset that "a little junk food will not hurt me." This is because some unhealthy foods can be addictive and are made in such a way as to cause craving which results in unreasonable indulgence in the unhealthy food. Unreasonable indulgence in an unhealthy food results in weight gain.

Be consistent in your effort to achieve good health. Get rid of everything around you that support your weight gain and restock your pantry and refrigerator with healthy foods.

II. Thinking Realistically and Profitably about Your Health as It Relates to Your Weight

Avoid seeing weight as a size issue. Weight that is outside a healthy range can have consequences that can be devastating. It can threaten one's activities, peace, comfort, and happiness. Some people who are overweight have diminished self esteem which adversely affects their relationships.

Anything that contributes to your weight gain threatens your good health as well. When your good health is threatened, your job or daily function is adversely affected. When your job is adversely affected, financial loss may result. Furthermore, increase in weight that is unchecked can result in a number of undesirable effects including disability directly or indirectly. Not only are you adversely affected by the consequences of excess weight, your family is negatively affected as well.

The measures you choose to implement to lose weight are important. There are right measures and wrong measures. Wrong measures can affect adversely your job, daily functions and the people you love.

When considering your weight, think ahead. You may be alright now but will that situation continue with reasonable certainty as years go by? Remind yourself through outcome projection journal that a precious reward of good health awaits you at the end of all your efforts. Let this be an incentive to go on when tempted to do otherwise; or when tempted not to care anymore.

III.   Lifestyle of Adhering to Healthy Choices

Healthy choices should be part of a daily commitment. Avoid weight loss measures that cannot be a permanent part of your life. These leave room for weight lost to be gained back thereby returning you to your starting weight. Lifestyle modification that results in a healthy weight serves a long term purpose and enables you to curb weight fluctuations. Inability to maintain a steady healthy weight can cause you to give up trying to be healthy and think that you are unable to succeed in this area of life.

Find healthier choices for everything that contributes to your weight gain. Remember, for everything you eat that contributes to your weight gain there is a healthier alternative. Believe me, some healthier alternatives can taste really good and leave you with no guilty feeling or a payback with excess weight or ill health. Make choosing and eating the right foods a priority daily.

Also, test or evaluate weight loss measures with regard to how they affect your health even when they keep you consistently thin. Remember that healthy choices enrich various areas of life. You can positively influence the important people in your life through your healthy choices.

Action Summary # 2

You have powerful tools at your disposal which can change your health and life for the better. These powerful tools are: choice, determination and commitment. If you determine to maintain your body appropriately, commit to this appropriate maintenance of the body and adhere to choices that move you in this direction. You will become healthy and maintain good health.

Strive for a healthy body, it is not automatic. It requires conscious and appropriate thoughts and actions. The maintenance of a good and healthy weight is part of maintaining good health. The actions that allow you to have good weight also allow you to have good health. You also need to maintain the right weight in the right way. Unhealthy means of weight loss are unacceptable as they lead to ill health in spite of lost weight.

When you maintain a good weight, you will not develop diseases that are precipitated by excess weight. Avoidance of diseases will significantly enhance your health.

Chapter Three

Healthy Thoughts for Healthy Weight

Healthy living and healthy weight go together. Some patients discuss their weight loss efforts with me while others seek counsel for products in the pharmacy that can help them lose weight. Weight control has multiple benefits. It is important, therefore, that you maintain a healthy weight before any sickness. The difference is that if you maintain your ideal weight before you have to, you will be healthy and happy and your effort will be abundantly rewarded. If you lose weight while sick, you will have your sickness to worry about in addition to your weight until your weight and health improve.

Your mind-set is important as far as your weight is concerned. The way you think about your weight and the way you talk about your weight may determine your success or failure in achieving a healthy weight. There are healthy and unhealthy ways to perceive your weight. Healthy ways of perceiving your weight propel you to positive, profitable action. An unhealthy way of perceiving your weight, on the other hand, may demoralize you. It might make you eat unhealthy foods for comfort which complicates healthy weight efforts.

Unhealthy weight ought to be seen as a detour on your road to a healthy lifestyle. If you drive a car or ride in a car, you must have come across a big sign at some point. The big sign usually says one word. That one word is "Detour." Detour on the road simply means that you need an immediate change of direction. You are still able to get to your destination. However, you have to make a change from your normal route to get to your destination. This is not a desirable experience but it happens in life anyway. No one who sees the detour sign says, "I will no longer get to my destination because I see a detour sign." Realizing that you have gained more weight than you need to be healthy is like your body putting out a health sign for you. This health sign tells you that you need a 'health detour' that will get your weight to a healthy destination which you deserve and are well able to attain. It does not call for you to quit trying to have a healthy weight or a healthy lifestyle.

Talk yourself into helpful actions that will benefit your weight. Remain positive about obtaining and maintaining a healthy weight. Instead of saying "I am fat now" simply say "I need a health detour now," and get started on a "health detour."

Seven Do's and Don'ts about Your Weight

I will discuss seven things you should do about your weight that will be beneficial to you and seven things you should not do because they will impair your progress.

Seven Do's about Your Weight

(1) Do remember that your weight is not written in stone

(2) Do remember that you have the ability to change your weight

(3) Do remember that you have to do something differently to change your weight

(4) Do remember that weight responds to lifestyle changes

(5) Do remember that a good change for the better is a change that you can commit to and repeat daily

(6) Do remember that a healthy weight results in a healthy body

(7) Do remember that you, yes you, can attain a healthy weight

Seven Don'ts about Your Weight

(1) Do not defeat yourself by saying that you are fat (or big) and that you cannot help it

(2) Do not say that good weight does not work for you

(3) Do not protect habits that make you gain weight

(4) Do not insist on eating a food item that make you gain weight

(5) Do not say that there is something that you cannot give up even for weight

(6) Do not postpone making healthy choices and changes that lead to healthy weight

(7) Do not say that you have failed before in your healthy weight efforts and so need not try again

Measuring and Keeping Track of Your Weight

For some reason, extra weight creeps up on people. You may be unable to say when your weight started to shift from ideal weight to an unhealthy weight. All of a sudden your clothes do not fit and you need a new wardrobe. Since prevention is a powerful tool for success against ill health, we need to keep track of our weight in different ways. Evaluating your weight by using one parameter alone, such as the reading on the scale, might be inadequate. You can miss out on pertinent information that is not reflected on the scale, for instance. Using multiple means to keep track of your weight allows you to have a balanced idea of your weight and your weight loss progress. My athletic experiences and exposure to patient situations allow me to understand that the weight on the scale alone is not all there is to weight.

Keeping Track of Your Weight

There are seven important ways that you can monitor your weight:

(1) Monitoring weight by weighing one's self on the scale
(2) Monitoring weight by measuring one's waist circumference
(3) Observing one's size in the mirror
(4) Taking note of the way your clothes fit
(5) Taking note of the onset of continued desire to eat larger portions of food than usual

(6) Adjusting weight downward if there is family history of Type II diabetes, premature heart disease, high blood pressure, or high cholesterol

(7) Monitoring weight by calculating the body mass Index (BMI)

(1) Monitoring Weight by Weighing Yourself on the Scale

Visiting the good old scale is still in style. Until the desired weight is achieved, it will be helpful to weigh yourself about four times a week and note the result. One may weigh oneself in the morning at about the same time for consistency. The attitude to this weighing should not be a fear of obtaining a demerit if the weight does not fall within a desired range. Basically, the scale should be viewed as a guide to help one determine what the next step should be towards achieving the desired outcome in weight.

Remember, if you are working out and gaining muscle you will look more toned but you may not see a dramatic reduction in weight for a while. You might even weigh more initially. Do not worry about the extra weight you notice if it is due to increased muscle mass because increased muscle mass has benefits towards obtaining a healthy body. This is why monitoring weight in several ways is appropriate.

(2) Monitoring Weight by Measuring Your Waist Circumference

Use a tape to measure your waist circumference. Breathe out and then take the measurement right after breathing out. Measure the area just above the hip. Having a lot of fat around the waist predisposes you to Type II diabetes and heart disease.

Waist Circumference Values to be Aware of

Increased risk for Type II diabetes and heart disease is associated with the following values:

Waist circumference for men, greater than 40 inches and,

Waist circumference for women, greater than 35 inches

If your waist circumference is small, you can skip the waist circumference measurement.

(3) Observing Your Size in the Mirror

You may say, "I have an idea of my size, why should I stand in front of the mirror just to observe my size?" Observing yourself in the mirror sounds basic but it is important. Observing oneself in the mirror is a weight monitoring opportunity that can easily be overlooked, taken for granted or ignored altogether. Observing yourself in front of a full length mirror with the intention of noting any significant change in your weight is a good thing. Again, this is a pointer to what to do next in the process of achieving the desired weight. It should not be viewed as an examination with a passing or failing grade in mind. This is useful for everyone.

Some people even when they observe themselves in the mirror, stop paying attention to the size they see after sometime. They look in the mirror to ensure that their clothes fit well or that their make-up is even or that their ties are neatly in place. Weight could get completely excluded from consideration as far as appearance goes, until sickness reminds someone of the omission. Observing your weight in front of a full length mirror is particularly important if you are working out and gaining some muscles. Muscles weigh more than fat. Therefore, if you have lost fat and gained muscle, your loss of fat might not be immediately apparent from your weight on the scale. The mirror, however, will allow you to see that you have lost some fat.

(4) Taking Note of the Way Your Clothes Fit

Being aware of how your clothes fit also sounds basic. It is, however, pertinent to weight evaluation. People have less time to prepare for outings due to busier schedules. The last thing a lot of people want to worry about is how snug their clothes fit. If the clothing item fits reasonably, they will continue with their day's schedule. If the clothing item becomes too tight, they will head out to purchase new clothes. Before rushing off to buy the next larger sized clothing, consider the type of adjustment you need to make to maintain a healthy weight. If you have lost weight, on the other hand, you will notice that from the way your clothes fit as well.

(5) Monitor Continued Desire to Eat Larger Portions of Food than Usual

Use caution when satisfying constant desire to eat. Do not allow your food portions to continue to increase and get larger and larger over time. On the contrary, decrease your portion size if you increase the frequency with which you eat. Ensure that you have an idea of the amount of fiber that you are taking in.

(6) Adjusting Weight Downward When There Is Family History of Type II Diabetes, Premature Heart Disease, High Blood Pressure, or High Cholesterol

If you have a family history of Type II diabetes, premature heart disease, high blood pressure, or high cholesterol, it will be best for you to make an effort to stay within your ideal weight. You cannot control your family history but you can minimize the risk factors for diseases in your family. One way to do this is by maintaining a healthy weight.

(7) Monitoring Weight by Calculating the Body Mass Index (BMI)

Body mass index (BMI) is used to assess overweight and obesity. It is a useful indicator of body fat for most people. It is important to remember that athletes who are well trained have a higher BMI due to increased muscles and not increased fat.

BMI Calculation

BMI can be calculated for weight measured in kilograms (kg) and height in meters (m)

OR

BMI can be calculated for weight measured in pounds (Ibs) and height in inches (in.)

BMI Calculation: Example I

BMI for weight measured in kilograms (kg) and height in meters (m)

BMI = Weight (kg) divided by height (m) that is squared

BMI = Weight (kg)/ [height (m)]2

Note: Centimeter (cm) to meter (m) conversion; 100 cm = 1 m

For someone who weighs 60 kg with a height of 160 cm or 1.60 m the BMI will be calculated as follows:

BMI = 60 (kg)/[1.60 (m)]2

 = 60 /2.56 = 23.44

BMI = 23.44

BMI Calculation: Example II

BMI for weight measured in pounds (Ibs) and height in inches (in.)

BMI = Weight (Ibs) divided by height (in.) that is squared and the answer from this is multiplied by 703

BMI = Weight (Ibs)/[Height (in.)]2 x 703

Note: Inches (in.) to feet (ft) conversion; 12 ins. is equal to 1ft

For someone who weighs 170 Ibs with a height of 6 ft 2 in. or 74 in. the BMI will be calculated as follows:

BMI = 170 (Ibs)/[74 (in.)]2 x 703

= 170/5476 x703 = 21.82

BMI = 21.82

BMI up to 25 is overweight and up to 30 is obese.

Body Mass Index for Children and Teens

For children and teens, BMIs compare their heights and weights against growth charts. The growth chart takes into consideration their sex and age. BMI percentile is used for children, from 2 to 19 years old.

For children and teens, 5th percentile to less than the 85th percentile is healthy weight.

Action Summary # 3

Begin to think appropriately for a healthy weight. The best thing to do is to avoid thoughts that defeat you and make you give up in your efforts towards good weight. You, yes you, can have a healthy weight. No matter the reason why you are not maintaining your ideal weight, your weight can change. Remember, always, that your weight is not written in stone.

There are various ways to keep track of your weight. For weight measurement use as many of the weight measuring or evaluating tools as are applicable and useful to you. When you keep track of your weight, it is best to see the weight you observe as a call for profitable action that will help you to reach your goal.

Avoid seeing your weight as having a failing grade or a demerit. A weight that is outside your desired goal is a health detour. It is not the end of the journey to your destination. You will still get to your destination as far as your weight is concerned. You just need to go in a different direction. This means that you will do a few things differently. You will need to include some things in your life and remove some things from your life. Achieving your ideal weight will not happen overnight or even in the first week. Be patient as you pursue your weight goal. As long as you are adhering to the right actions which include making the right changes, you are on the right track. The most important thing in the pursuit of a healthy weight is progress. Pursue progress rather than overnight success.

As long as you are making progress, success will eventually be achieved.

Chapter Four

Food Considerations

While medications play important roles in our health, they should not take the place of nourishing foods. Eating the wrong foods may result in deleterious health effects that may require treatment with medications. I strongly believe in knowing as much as possible about what I eat and so have paid close attention to different foods over the years. My husband teases me and calls me a food Czar sometimes. He lets me know that my food choices for our home and what I choose at restaurants get featured in the news, years after I have chosen them, as giving health a boost. In preparing to counsel patients as a pharmacist on vitamins, I also learn what foods contain.

I also pay close attention to what foods patients who have to be on medications need to eat or avoid for better health or for medical condition resolution. I carefully examine various food labels and even more so with the writing of this book. Some of the information on foods is required while others are volunteered to encourage people to eat certain foods. Some effects of the food that people eat stand out, while others are concealed.

Even when we do not realize it everything we eat either moves us in the direction of enhanced health or diminished health. There is really no middle ground when it comes to food. What we eat is either healthy or unhealthy. Many of us tend to eat what we like and desire. Some of our desires need to be re-evaluated to keep up with our health needs. You can like certain things that can turn out to be a hindrance to good health. Some foods taste so good and yet are so bad for your health. Unfortunately, taste alone cannot be the only consideration for the types of foods and snacks that we eat. What we put into our bodies is manifested in our health. Sooner or later your body will update you on how you are eating with regard to your weight and health.

Natural Foods

It is a well known epidemiologic fact that some diseases such as colorectal cancer and cardiovascular diseases are very prevalent in the United States and other western industrialized countries. Such diseases are rare in less industrialized countries where the diet comprises natural unprocessed foods that are rich in fiber and healthy fats.

In November, 2010, I visited my sister in Pennsylvania. As a practicing physician my sister, Dr. Eby Ufondu, impacts the lives of her patients by helping them make healthy life choices. She goes beyond the call of duty. She not only cares about healthy bodies, she cares about healthy minds as well; which in turn enhances overall health. I always encourage people to eat natural foods. I was delighted about her healthy eating habits. She is putting into practice what she recommends to her patients.

Wrong Actions that Can Send You to the Emergency Room

Eating the right foods and snacks is part of the right and proper maintenance of your body. Eating the wrong foods and snacks is part of the wrong maintenance of your body. Wrong maintenance of the body results in problems with our health.

I know some people who were told after a visit to the emergency room that what they were eating caused the medical emergency that brought them to the hospital. Some of these people are my acquaintances. I have also interviewed people who suffered medical emergencies that were traced back to food.

Some people depend on the fast food restaurants for a lot of their meals. If you are unable to prepare your own food to take to work or activities, you may depend on fast foods. If you enjoy a generous amount of hamburger and fries for your lunch every day from the fast food restaurants, you may end up most likely in the emergency room over time with a heart attack. The excess amount of fat and the carbohydrate with high glycemic index from this type of food is not good for your health.

If you are a potato chip lover and indulge in the consumption of a medium to large bag of potato chips every day, you can end up some day in the emergency room in at least a hypertensive state. The extra salt and fat in potato chips are not good for your health. Other habits that adversely affect your health include the daily consumption of generous amount of pastries for breakfast and sugary pies for desert. These can increase weight and adversely affect health.

The Biggest Weight Loss Hidden Obstacle

Some people want to lose weight as part of living a healthy lifestyle. They put in efforts but are unable to see result. Avoid falling prey to hidden obstacles. The single biggest sabotage of weight loss is the adherence to misconceptions manifested in wrong choices. Soda or sugary drink, for instance is a wrong beverage choice; a hidden weight loss obstacle. We cannot seem to get away from the call of the pounds and the call for belly size extension through sodas. We are served sodas at parties and other gatherings. We are surrounded by soda machines. The groceries and gas stations entice us with big savings on sodas. Even our favorite games commercials call for soda consumption.

If all the sale opportunities inviting us to indulge in sodas are not enough temptation to expand our waistlines, the fast food restaurants generously offer us the 'grand slam' of soda consumption opportunity; the supersized, extra large soda drinks. The supersized soda sells for just a few cents more than large soda drinks that come with the meals. We are usually invited to take advantage of the soda deals. At the moment, usually, it would look like we are getting something good; after all, we are getting a lot of beverage at a great price. We cannot allow the commercial promotion of sodas to influence our beverage choice. Sodas are not part of healthy drinks that are recommended for good health and weight.

Love and Consumption of Sodas: A Pitfall?

Let us consider a can of soft drink or soda. It contains about 145 calories which is mainly from sugar in the form of high fructose corn syrup. If you drink four cans of soft drinks per day for instance, you will consume, by so doing, the equivalent of about 40 teaspoonfuls of table sugar in one day from your drinks alone. A lot of people will not consider it appropriate to consume 40 teaspoonfuls of sugar in one day and yet a lot of people will drink at least four cans of soda in one day or its equivalent. Soft drinks rapidly boost the blood sugar and if cans or glasses of soft drink are taken daily it will eventually lead to abdominal fat, obesity and type II diabetes. This is why it is very important that you consider where anything you eat or drink fits in terms of a healthy diet and your overall health long term.

Diet Sodas

Some people are determined to stay hydrated through the consumption of sodas. They know that the extra sugar in the sodas or soft drinks is not good for them. So they reach for diet sodas. Diet sodas are sweetened with artificial sweeteners which are calorie-free and go by various names. These drinks over time can still lead to weight gain. The weight loss from diet drinks might not be permanent.

Other Beverages

I will review some of the other beverages that are available. I will then discuss beverages recommended for frequent consumption.

How about Fruit Punches and Beverages Ending in –'ade'?

Fruit punches, lemonades, orangeades, and beverages such as these are now abundant. These types of beverages are also discouraged as much as sodas are discouraged. They are not recommended for frequent consumption. If you find yourself consuming glasses of sugary drinks daily, that could signal trouble for your health and weight sooner or later.

Soda or Soft Drink Alternative

It will be profitable for you to choose an alternative to sugary drinks. A good alternative is water with fresh lemon squeezed into it without added sugar.

Daily Hydration: What Beverage Is Best for You?

There are numerous beverages available today. There is a stiff competition among the beverages. In spite of modern day competition for beverages, one beverage comes out on top and is recommended for daily consumption and hydration. The very best way to keep your body hydrated on a daily basis is by drinking plenty of good old water. I guess you could say that water is the king of all beverages. Water is an inexpensive way to keep hydrated. The amount of water recommended each day for women is about 11 to 12 cups and for men it is about 15 cups. This amount of water per day includes water in healthy watery soups and fresh foods. Obtaining water from fresh foods and healthy watery soups is a simple way of meeting the water requirement. It is very important for parents to remember that all children both younger and older ones need plenty of water also. Some people tend to think that children can drink whatever makes them happy or what they have adopted from commercials as their favorite drink. It is time to step away from this kind of misconception. Young children should be made aware of the importance of water to their health.

Green Tea

Plain green tea with no sugars added to it is good for you. It has a lot of flavonoids. It also has antioxidants. About two cups of green tea a day is beneficial in addition to a lot of water. When you take plenty of water and some green tea, you may go to the restroom more frequently. Plan ahead and make room for the restroom breaks.

Fruit Juices

Fruit juices include but are not limited to; orange juice, grapefruit juice, grape juice, mango juice, cranberry juice, pineapple juice, and apple juice. Fruit juices which contain 100% juice have majority of the nutrients in the fruit. The fruit juices are also fortified with some nutrients. Orange juice has calcium fortified option. When shaken well before each serving, an eight-ounce glass of calcium fortified orange juice, for instance, provides about 30% of daily calcium and 100% of daily vitamin C. Orange juice and other fruit juices provide more energy for the body than the fruits. It is good to remember this and so adjust for the additional calorie from fruit juice compared to the fruit. An eight-ounce glass of orange juice per day is beneficial.

All natural, 100% grape juice has a lot of antioxidants. It provides a lot of calories to the body and so can be limited to four ounces per day or one-half of a cup. Other 100% juices can also be limited to four to eight ounces per day depending on the calorie content.

Vegetable Juices

Vegetable juices may not contain a lot of calories. When considering vegetable juices, pay attention to the sodium content.

Sports Drink

Sports drinks are helpful when people have lost some fluids. Instances where sports drinks are beneficial include the use of sports drinks by athletes who are involved in high level of physical activities which make them sweat. Sports drinks are also good for people who have lost a lot of fluid due to vomiting or diarrhea.

Milk

Milk is a great source of calcium. It is usually fortified with vitamin D. Vitamin D enhances calcium absorption. If you are taking milk which contains calcium and vitamin D, choose 1% milk or skim milk. Lactose-free milk is available for people who have lactose intolerance. Some of the milk choices are now fortified with calcium and they have as much as 50% of the daily value for calcium per cup. Two cups of the calcium fortified milk provide you with100% of the daily requirement. Therefore, if you drink a cup of the fortified milk and use a second cup with a whole grain cereal on the same day, for instance, you will obtain the daily recommended amount of calcium. This will be helpful for teenagers who are undergoing rapid growth. It will help them to maintain strong bones.

Remember to shake the milk well before you serve it, so that you can obtain the needed nutrients in each cup of milk. This applies to other fortified liquids also. Shake them well, always, before serving them.

Action Summary # 4

Eat always, foods that enhance your health. What will be helpful today is to go ahead and get rid of all the unhealthy foods around you. Free your refrigerators, pantries, cabinets, and cars of all unhealthy foods and snacks. Find healthy alternatives to all the unhealthy foods and snacks that you eat daily. Mentally place every food in one of two categories. These two categories are: your daily foods (eaten every day) and occasional foods (eaten only once in a while). Eat educed portion of the occasional foods.

Discontinue eating habits that will cause you to have a medical emergency. Start today and switch from drinking sodas or soft drinks to water. Avoid diet soft drink or zero calorie soft drink. They are not good for you over time. Aim at about seven (of eight-ounce) glasses of water and about two glasses of the other healthy beverages a day. You can drink one glass of 100% orange juice (one eight-ounce cup) and one-half glass of 100% purple grape juice a day. You can also have one glass of 100% apple juice and one cup of green tea a day. You can have them on different days. One glass of calcium fortified 1% or low-fat milk a day is also helpful. Milk is very important for young children and teenagers.

Chapter Five

Healthy Diets

Healthy diets provide useful nutrition that is needed daily by the body. They also enhance health and decrease disease risk.

Important Components of a Healthy Diet

For optimal health, everything that a person consumes on a regular basis should be part of a planned balanced diet. It is a good idea to determine how to include in your daily diet healthy food choices. I will discuss some foods that are components of a healthy diet.

Carbohydrates

Food like 100% whole grain oats (oatmeal) is one of the best carbohydrate sources. One serving of 100% whole oats (one-half cup) contains four grams of fiber which is about 15% of the daily required fiber. It has zero sodium. Whole grain bread, such as 100% whole wheat bread, is also a good carbohydrate source. When you eat 100% whole wheat bread, reducing the portion is very important to avoid unnecessary weight gain.

Fruits and vegetables are great sources of carbohydrates. Beans are excellent sources of carbohydrates. They have very low glycemic index and so do not lead to a spike in blood sugar. This is beneficial.

Proteins

Nuts and beans are excellent sources of plant protein. Examples of nuts include but are not limited to almonds and walnuts. Examples of beans include but are not limited to navy beans, black-eyed peas, black beans, and kidney beans

Other good sources of protein include fish, eggs, and poultry (which are examples of animal protein). I will strongly recommend consumption of clean fish such as wild caught salmon and orange roughy. Poultry such as turkey and chicken are good protein sources and their saturated fat content can be low. Skinless poultry is best.

Dairy

For dairy needs, use skim milk or 1% milk and avoid whole milk. It is necessary to avoid whole milk because of the generous amount of saturated fat contained in whole milk. Use Lactose-free milk if you need it. Also limited amount of string mozzarella cheese made with 2 % milk can contribute to dairy need. It has 50 calories each. Another dairy product that is available is plain low-fat or fat-free yogurt as well as lactose-free yogurt.

Yogurt

Choose yogurt cautiously. I reviewed extensively the labels of various yogurts. When choosing yogurt, avoid those that are packed with saturated fat. Some regular (full-fat) yogurts contain in a seven to eight ounce serving size saturated fat ranging from five grams to sixteen grams. Some Greek yogurts have up to sixteen grams of saturated fat for these serving sizes. The daily recommended amount of saturated fat is twenty grams or less. A yogurt with sixteen grams of saturated fat has already in one serving 80% of the daily recommended amount of saturated fat for a 2,000 calorie diet. There are several yogurts to choose from. Avoid any food with high saturated fat content. Foods high in saturated fat will increase blood cholesterol and result in heart diseases.

Choose plain low-fat or non-fat yogurt. When choosing low-fat yogurt, avoid those with artificial sweeteners and artificial flavors. Avoid, also, those with a long list of artificial ingredients. Plain yogurt options with very few ingredients and whose ingredients are natural are best. You have the choice of Greek plain low-fat or non-fat yogurt. You also can choose regular plain low-fat or non-fat yogurt.

In choosing yogurt read the label and check the amount of following items:

- Calories
- Calcium
- Carbohydrate (total)
- Cholesterol
- Protein

- Saturated Fat (You need zero or very low saturated fat content)
- Sodium
- Sugar (You need low sugar content)
- Vitamin D (This is helpful for calcium absorption)

Pros for Plain Non-Fat Greek Yogurt

- They have lower sodium content than regular plain non-fat yogurt; 50 to 65 milligrams for about a six ounce serving. This is better for blood pressure control.
- They have higher protein content than regular plain non-fat yogurt; 15 to 18 grams for about a six ounce serving. More protein results in better satiation so you feel fuller for a longer time.
- They have lower total carbohydrates content than regular plain non-fat yogurt; about seven grams for a six ounce serving. This results in lower blood glucose levels and less chance of weight increase.
- They have lower sugar content than regular plain non-fat yogurt; about seven grams for a six ounce serving. This results in lower blood glucose levels and less chance of weight increase.
- Some brands have zero cholesterol content in a six ounce serving. This is better for the heart.
- They have less calorie content than plain non-fat yogurt; about 100 calories for a six ounce serving.

Cons for Plain Non-Fat Greek Yogurt

- They have lower calcium content than regular plain non-fat yogurt; about 20% of daily required amount of calcium for a 2,000 calorie diet in a six ounce serving. This is not as good for the bones as regular plain non-fat yogurt. You can take calcium fortified milk with them. Some calcium fortified milk options have in one serving or cup, 50% of daily value of calcium for a 2,000 calorie diet

- They do not have any listed amount of vitamin D (calcium absorption is not facilitated with it). You can take them with milk that has vitamin D in it.

- They do not have any vitamin A and thus not beneficial for vision.

Pros for Regular Plain Non-Fat Yogurt

- They have higher calcium content than plain Greek non-fat yogurt; about 30% of daily recommended calcium for a 2,000 calorie diet. They are better for bone health than plain Greek non-fat yogurt.

- They have lower cholesterol than plain Greek non-fat yogurt; less than five milligrams per six ounce serving. This results in lower risk of heart disease.

- They have in a six ounce serving 25% of daily required amount of vitamin D for a 2,000 calorie diet. This will enhance calcium absorption for healthier bone.

- They have in a six ounce serving 10% of daily required amount of vitamin A for a 2,000 calorie diet. They enhance vision.

Cons for Regular Plain Non-Fat Yogurt

- They have higher sodium content than Greek yogurt (more than double the amount); about 120 to 140 milligrams of sodium in a six ounce serving. There is more concern for blood pressure control with them than with plain Greek non-fat yogurt. Reduce sodium from other sources with these yogurts.
- They have less protein than Greek yogurt; about nine grams in a six ounce serving. They keep you less full. If you eat this yogurt, add healthy protein to it. Eating it with 12 almonds will add about three grams of protein to it.
- They have higher total carbohydrate content than Greek yogurt (more than double the amount); about 19 grams in a six ounce serving. This will lead to higher blood glucose levels and greater chance of weight increase.
- They have higher sugar content than Greek yogurt; about 12 grams in a six ounce serving. This will lead to higher blood glucose levels and increased chance of weight gain.

The Greek yogurt has more benefits overall. Whichever one of the two yogurt types you choose, make adjustment in your other foods for what is unfavorably high or unfavorable low in the yogurt. This will enable you to maintain a healthy balance in your daily foods. Daily consumption of one serving of plain low-fat or non-fat yogurt is profitable for weight control. You can add fresh fruits and limited amount of nuts, such as almonds, to the yogurt for better taste.

Organic Yogurt

Organic yogurt is also available. It is made without the use of synthetic hormones and antibiotics. It is not associated with generous pesticide exposure. The package label will indicate if the yogurt is organic. Buy organic when that is possible.

Healthy Proteins, Fats, Oils, and Omega-3 Fatty Acids

Proteins, fat, and oils are available from various sources. It is important to choose them carefully. I will discuss these briefly as well as omega-3 fatty acids.

Unhealthy and Healthy Proteins

Unhealthy Protein Sources

Unhealthy protein can adversely affect your health. Maintain caution and avoid eating any kind of processed meat in spite of their numerous sources today. Processed meats that you need to avoid include bacon, cold cuts (cold cooked meats that are sliced) like processed turkey slices, and other processed meats.

Some people want to eat healthy and for lunch they chose a sandwich with processed meat. The processed meat automatically renders such lunches unhealthy. Be sure to eat sandwiches with meats from healthy natural sources for your lunch or dinner. Avoid any type of fried meat.

Proteins and Amino Acids

Proteins contain amino acids which are used as building blocks for making new proteins by the body. Proteins from animal sources such as fish and poultry tend to contain all the amino acids that the body needs to make new proteins. This is not the case with plant proteins.

Healthy Proteins

Plant proteins are highly recommended as top choice for healthy protein. Plant proteins, however, do not contain all the amino acids needed for making new proteins in the body. Fish and poultry will help to add some amino acids to the body in addition to amino acids from plant protein. Eating protein-rich foods from a wide range of sources each day will be a good option for people who are vegetarians. Broadening the sources of plant protein will ensure a wider range of amino acids from plants.

Unhealthy and Healthy Fats

Unhealthy Fats

Unhealthy fats are those fats that are labeled as partially hydrogenated oil. They are the trans fat. Fats sources which contain trans fat are bad for your health. They lower HDL which is the good cholesterol. They also increase LDL which is the bad cholesterol. They increase your chance of developing heart disease. It is recommended that no more than 20 calories per day should come from trans fat for a 2,000 calorie per day need. Your goal should be to avoid trans fat altogether in oils and eat foods free of trans fat.

Healthy Fats

Eat foods that contain healthy fats. Remember, butter is not part of a healthy diet. Consider using extra virgin olive oil in place of butter. If you must use butter, decrease the quantity to about one-fifth of the total amount needed; use 20% butter and 80% extra virgin olive oil. **Healthy fats increase HDL and decrease LDL.** Obtain dietary fats from healthy sources that contain polyunsaturated fat. These include nuts such as almonds and seeds.

Almonds: Noteworthy Nuts

Almonds are packed with nutrients. They have a lot of health benefits. They contain vitamin E (tocopherol) which is an antioxidant. One serving of almonds contains as much as 35% of the daily amount of vitamin E. They contain vitamin B2 (riboflavin). They also contain several minerals that help to facilitate the functions of the body. These minerals include calcium and iron. They also contain magnesium, manganese, copper, phosphorus, and zinc that benefit the body.

Eat healthy almonds. All natural raw almonds are very beneficial. They have no sodium or cholesterol and they also have lower calories than the almonds that have added ingredients. They also have about one gram of sugar per serving. Avoid salted almonds. Increased salt intake adversely affects blood pressure. Chocolate covered almonds should be avoided. They contain almost 10 times the amount of sugar contained in natural almonds. Their calorie content is much higher than those of natural raw almonds and this is not helpful as far as weight is concerned. When almonds are covered with chocolate, eating them even in small quantity could contribute to weight gain. Increased weight that is not addressed could increase the risk of type II diabetes.

Reduce the portion of your almonds so that you can enjoy their health benefits without gaining weight (if they cause you to gain weight). One serving of almonds is about 24 nuts or one-fourth cup. The serving size of the almonds in terms of the number of nuts per serving will be on the package label. Eat about 12 almonds and eat them about three to four days a week. If you eat 12 almonds, that will be one-half of a serving. You can have six almonds twice a day or 12 almonds once a day. You can also use almonds as protein in place of meat or use reduced meat portion as a result of adding some almonds to your meal.

Healthier Oils

Use healthier oils containing unsaturated fat such as extra virgin and virgin olive oils. Do not indulge in oil even when they are healthy. You can use one and one-half teaspoonful of extra virgin olive oil and one-fourth to one-half teaspoonful of black pepper on salad in place of fatty unhealthy salad dressings that sabotage your healthy eating.

Olive Oils Basics

Olive oils have different labeling on them. Olive oil is made by crushing olives. After harvesting, the olives are crushed and then put in a press to extract the olive oil. The olive oil, then, is marketed. Extra virgin and virgin olive oils are more natural than the processed olive oils. They are not chemically refined. The Extra virgin olive oils are usually stored in dark bottles. Storing olive oil in a dark place or cabinet is beneficial. The olive oils should have dates on them. It is best if they are used within one year for maximum health benefits.

The different types of olive oils are as follows;

(I) Extra virgin olive oil: The extra virgin oil tastes the best of all the olive oils. They are the highest quality of olive oil. They have great odor as well.

(II) Virgin olive oil: The virgin olive oils taste good but not as good as the extra virgin olive oils. They have good odor.

(III)   Pure olive oil: The pure olive oil is a mixture of both chemically refined and virgin olive oil.

(IV)   Refined olive oil: This has only refined olive oils.

Omega-3 Fatty Acids

Omega-3 fatty acids help to reduce inflammation in the body. These inflammations include those that are capable of damaging blood vessels. Blood vessel damage results in heart disease. Omega-3 fatty acids are contained in fish and also in some nuts and seeds. Omega-3 fatty acids from fish contain two acids which are part of cell membranes. These are docosahexaenoic acid (DHA) and eicosapentaenoic acid (EPA). The human body cannot make from scratch omega-3 fatty acids including DHA and EPA. The body depends on food to get DHA and EPA. It is a very good idea to eat fish every week to supply your body with the DHA and the EPA that it needs for body functions. Cleaner fish such as wild caught salmon should be eaten. Ensure that there is indication that the fish is wild caught.

Non-fish sources of omega-3 fatty acid include walnuts, flaxseeds, and some vegetable oils such as flaxseed oil (a very important source of omega-3 fatty acid). This omega-3 fatty acid from plant source is known as Alpha-linolenic acid (ALA). The omega-3 fatty acids from fish have more beneficial effects on the heart than those from plant sources.

Benefits of Omega-3 Fatty Acids

Omega-3 fatty acid may have the following health benefits:

(1) May lower blood pressure

(2) May lower triglycerides

(3) May decrease blood clotting

(4) May boost mood

(5) May boost immunity

(6) Has beneficial effects on the skin

(7) Reduces blood vessel damage

(8) Reduces heart disease

Remember that the best source of omega-3 fatty acids is natural foods and not supplements.

Corn

A lot of the corns that are available are genetically modified to tolerate herbicide. Corn is also highly susceptible to pests which are controlled by the use of pesticides. There is a concern about the possibility of the presence of pesticides and herbicides in corn.

Organic corn unmodified and not treated with herbicides and pesticides can be eaten in limited amount. It also makes good popcorn snack if popped at home with small amount of olive oil and no butter.

Salt

Table salt is a combination of sodium and chloride (sodium chloride). Reducing salt intake is beneficial for good health. Everyone will benefit from taking no more than three-fourths of a teaspoonful of salt (1.8 grams or 1,800 milligrams) per day. Recommendation for someone who does not have disease states is about one teaspoonful (about 2.4 grams or 2,400 milligrams) per day.

Consuming a lot of sodium in the diet increases the amount of calcium that the body eliminates in the urine. It also increases the amount of calcium eliminated through sweating. When the body does not have enough calcium, it obtains calcium from bone thereby thinning the bones which will lead to osteoporosis. Beneficial calcium balance in the body is enhanced by reduced salt intake.

Gluten and Monosodium Glutamate (MSG)

What about Gluten?

Gluten is a protein found in grains such as wheat, barley, and rye. Common foods such as bread contain gluten. Some people believe that to be healthy and energetic you need a gluten-free diet. Gluten-free diet is not for everybody. It is necessary, however, for people with celiac disease or people who have adverse reactions due to gluten. If you are always tired while maintaining a healthy lifestyle or have unexpected symptoms such as gastrointestinal problems that affect your health adversely, consult your physician for evaluation.

MSG Caution

MSG is a flavor booster that is added to foods. Some people are allergic to MSG and so suffer from adverse reactions when they eat foods to which it is added. Food labels usually indicate if MSG is added to it. There are alternative flavors for foods that do not contain MSG.

Meal Treats and Healthy Meals

Whatever you eat or drink, whether you think much about it or not, belong to one of two critical groups of foods and beverages. These groups are:

(1) Occasional foods and beverages
(2) Daily foods and beverages

As soon as you can put everything you eat into one of the above groups in your mind, healthy eating will become easier for you.

Avoid indulging in what I call 'meal treats.' I will define meal treats as any type of food or beverage whose enticement include taste and enjoyment, which if taken on a daily basis will interfere with your good health, good weight and optimal functioning. Examples of meal treats are: pastries such as doughnuts, tarts, croissants, strudels, candies, pies, cakes, and regular ice cream.

Other examples are: baked potatoes, white bread, white rice, white flour pastas, French fries, butter, margarine, none whole grain pancakes, bacon, sausages, regular crust processed meat pizzas, fatty hamburgers, various fried foods, and fatty red meat Beverages in this category include soda, fruit punch, lemonade, orangeade, energy drink, and whole milk.

Some meal treats also contain unhealthy saturated fats. Meal treats should be removed from your daily diet. Eating them only twice in a month or less is best. Reduce the portion that you consume. Eat one-third to one-half of one serving. Monitor the extra calories gained from the meal treats and burn off those calories. Remember the health risks that are associated with the meal treats.

Healthy meals in contrast to meal treats help you to obtain your total calories per day appropriately. They also help you to obtain important nutrients. They help you to obtain your daily supply of healthy protein, carbohydrates, fat, fiber, vitamins, and minerals. These supply energy. They also contribute positively to the body's various metabolic processes.

Red Meat or Beef

There has been an ongoing discussion on whether red meat is good or bad for you. All that go into the cattle, from birth to the time it appears on your plate as beef, play an important role in this discussion. Red meat will be considered healthier if the cattle are grass-fed and if the grass used in their feeding is not doused (drenched) in pesticides, herbicides, and fungicides. The red meat will also be healthier if the cattle are not exposed to chemicals in other ways.

There are two types of red meat. There is the regular red meat which has generous amount of saturated fat. Saturated fat is the 'bad guy' type of fat. The second type of red meat is the lean red meat. Lean red meat has less saturated fat than regular red meat. Red meat is not recommended for daily consumption. Frequent or daily consumption of red meat, which contains generous amount of saturated fat and chemicals, can lead to some medical problems. This is the case, especially, where the cattle from which the beef is obtained are neither grass-fed nor naturally raised. When the term "naturally raised" is used for cattle it refers to some benefits. These include the fact that, except for parasite control, the cattle are raised without hormones and antibiotics.

 Medical conditions that may be associated with eating red meat daily include:

  (a) Increased risk of colorectal cancer
  (b) Increased risk of stroke
  (c) Increased risk of cardiovascular disease

Limit red meat consumption as suggested above. Lean red meat from grass-fed and naturally raised cattle is the preferred option.

The Biggest Eating Deception: A Mind Trap to Avoid

Some people want to have a healthy lifestyle. They agree that what we eat is important, however, they adopt an inadequate and deceptive point of view when it comes to healthy eating. These are people who believe that whatever you eat should be eaten in moderation. It sounds so good and reasonable but it is so inadequate and misleading as far as a healthy lifestyle is concerned. It is like sitting on the fence of healthy living.

When you believe this concept, you are partially acknowledging the importance of eating healthy while being unprepared to focus on eating only healthy foods. Eating whatever food comes your way is not good enough even if it is eaten in moderation. The implementation of this belief can greatly diminish your health and keep you from achieving a healthy weight. You will enjoy health benefits if you start eating the right foods and stop eating the wrong foods. If you eat bacon and doughnuts for breakfast every morning in moderation, hamburger and fries every afternoon for lunch in moderation, regular crust processed meat pizzas and pies every evening for dinner in moderation, you will greatly increase your risk of having a heart attack and Type II diabetes. You will also be unable to maintain a healthy weight. The type of foods that you chose to eat is critically important toward good health and weight. Whole hearted commitment is needed for desirable result in good health and weight.

The right amount of the right food, eaten the right way, is important for good health and weight. You may ask, "What do you mean by eating the right food the right way?" When chicken is broiled, for example, it will be healthy and will have minimal chance of causing symptoms such as acid reflux. Consider the same chicken if it is fried in oil rich in saturated fat, it will be unhealthy and will have increased chance of causing unhealthy symptoms such as heartburn.

Glycemic Index and Glycemic Load

Glycemic Index

Glycemic index is a means of classifying carbohydrate rich foods. Glycemic index values are obtained when carbohydrate rich foods are classified according to the speed and magnitude of their effects on blood glucose levels. It measures how rapidly glucose from food is absorbed.

A lot of meal treats have high glycemic index. They lead to a spike in blood glucose levels. Foods with low glycemic index when eaten, on the other hand, get converted to blood sugar slowly and so prevent a spike in blood sugar.

Glycemic Load

Glycemic load measures the total glucose in foods which can be absorbed. Foods which have low glycemic load will have less effect on blood glucose levels.

Baked Potato, White Rice, and White Spaghetti Issues

Glycemic index values of various foods are important. Baked potato, for instance, has a very high glycemic index. Eating a lot of it increases blood glucose level. If this is sustained, the risk of developing type II diabetes will increase; as well as weight gain and obesity. Type II diabetes in turn, increases the risk factors of developing some other disease states.

White rice has a high glycemic index. It is a staple food in some cultures and some people eat it almost every day. Portion of rice consumed is very important. Some people eat multiple servings of rice instead of one serving. This can elevate blood glucose level. If increased level of blood glucose is sustained, it could lead to type II diabetes. Consuming large amounts of white rice could also lead to weight gain and obesity, thereby increasing the risk of diseases that are affected by weight.

White spaghetti is another food with a high glycemic index. The major problem here is that some people eat three servings or more instead of one serving of spaghetti in one meal. This will increase blood glucose level and weight. These in turn would increase the risk of type II diabetes, obesity and some other diseases.

Suggestions for Foods such as Baked Potato, White Rice, and White Spaghetti

Baked Potato

If you eat baked potatoes you may want to decrease frequency of consumption to once a week and in reduced portion of about one-half of a serving. You can also switch to sweet potato. You can eat one-serving of sweet potatoes because portion size is important. Eat it with plenty of vegetables including broccoli about twice a week. It facilitates satiation and so enables people to eat less. Do not eat excessive amounts of sweet potatoes.

White Rice

People eat white rice for different reasons. Some people eat it for affordability. If you must eat white rice due to affordability or any other reason, you will need to make major adjustments to the rice to eat healthier. You will need to decrease the frequency of consumption to about three times a week. You will also need to reduce dramatically the portion of the rice that you eat.

It will be beneficial to prepare it in combination with very low glycemic index foods. You can use the combination that I call "legume tri-mix; high fiber." This means that for every cup of rice that you prepare, you will add three cups of foods such as black-eye peas or beans and two cups of mixed vegetables; such as green beans and sweet carrots or any other mixed vegetable of your choice. So you will eat black-eye peas (or beans), mixed vegetables and rice in the ratio of 3:2:1. This means that you will consume one-sixth of the amount of rice that you would have otherwise. You will make up the potion size with the high fiber components of the foods. These are also low in fat and are cholesterol-free.

You need to prepare the beans or peas for cooking. First you sort them in a large tray to remove those that are spoilt as well as any foreign body. Then wash them. Next soak them if it is dried beans. Black-eyed peas and lentils do not need soaking before they are cooked unless they cause bloating for you.

You can soak one pound (two cups) of beans in eight cups of water overnight or for about seven hours. You then discard the water, rinse the beans, and cook them in fresh water. Soaking instructions can also be found on the package label. If you have limited time, instead of soaking overnight use the quick soaking method. For a quick soaking option, sort and wash them. Boil eight cups of water in a pot and add the washed beans. Boil for another five minutes and set it aside for about one hour. After one hour, discard the water. Rinse about twice before cooking in fresh water. This will help the beans not to cause discomfort in form of gas or bloating. After soaking the beans it may be necessary to reduce the water for cooking it by about one cup if firmer texture is desired.

Recipes for Legume Tri-Mix; High Fiber (Black-Eyed Peas, Mixed Vegetables and Rice)

Ingredients;

- 3 cups of black-eyed peas
- 2 cups of mixed vegetables
- 1 cups of rice
- 1 cups of chopped onions
- 1 and ½ cups of cooked deviled shrimp (12 ounces)
- 2 baked salmon fillets (eight ounces) cut into chunks
- 4 teaspoonfuls of extra virgin olive oil
- 4 teaspoonfuls of seasoned salt divided in four
- ¾ teaspoonful of basil
- ¾ teaspoonful of garlic powder
- ½ teaspoonful of nutmeg
- ½ teaspoonful of curry powder
- ½ teaspoonful of black pepper
- ¼ teaspoonful of crushed red pepper
- ½ cup of water

First bring one cup of water to a boil in a small pot and add to it one teaspoonful of seasoned salt. Pour the washed mixed vegetables into it, mix well. Remove from heat, drain the water and set aside. Cook the cup of rice in two cups of water with one teaspoonful of seasoned salt, until the water dries up or according to package instructions. The rice is ready in 18 to 20 minutes. Then set it aside. Wash the sorted black-eyed peas twice, then rinse and cook them in five cups of water with one teaspoonful of salt until tender and set aside. It could take 60 minutes or longer to cook. Start checking it after 45 minutes to see if it can be crushed easily. Unlike the quick dinners in Chapter Nine of this book, beans and peas are not quick meals unless you cook the beans or peas ahead of time.

Do not fry the food. In a large frying pan add the water (one-half cup) and bring to a boil. Then add the chopped onions and stir frequently until tender and very slightly brown (about 10 minutes). You can cover it for about five minutes. Do not allow the onions to get scorched. Add the remaining teaspoonful of seasoned salt and stir well. Add basil leaves, nutmeg, curry powder, black pepper, red pepper and garlic; mix well. Add the olive oil and mix well also. Cook for five minutes, stirring frequently. Then add the shrimps and salmon. Continue to stir frequently for about five minutes. Add the mixed vegetables and mix well. Add the cooked black-eyed peas and rice and mix well also; the rice and peas being added should be at least warm. Cover and turn off heat. Remove from heat after about three minutes or as soon as the mixture is hot. Be sure not to overcook the vegetables. Ensure that the green vegetables are still green. This serves six to eight people.

Other Types of Legumes Including Beans, Beas and Lentils with Chicken

You can substitute any other legumes of your choice for black-eyed peas. You can then follow the rest of the recipe and adjust where necessary to taste. You can also follow the recipe and substitute skinless broiled chicken pieces for shrimps. Vegetarians could use mushrooms instead of shrimp or chicken.

Another Type of Rice

Whole grain wild rice can be used instead of white rice as a healthier option. Portion control is important even when wild rice is being consumed.

Spaghetti

If you eat spaghetti, reduce portion to one serving. Also reduce frequency of consumption to about once a week. You can substitute any legumes dinner of your choice for a spaghetti dinner about twice a week. You can also make the spaghetti with mixed vegetable, mushrooms and onions in a ratio of 1:1:1:1. This will reduce your spaghetti portion to one-fourth in one serving of the food or one-half of a cup of the food. The rest of the portion will be made up with mixed vegetables mushrooms and onions.

You can also use this ratio to prepare high fiber pasta that is now available. These high fiber white pastas have six grams of fiber in a two ounce serving.

Action Summary # 5

Eat healthy carbohydrates such as 100% whole grain old fashioned oats (oatmeal). Also add 100% whole wheat bread to your diet. Limit the quantity of bread that you eat. Avoid white bread and white dinner rolls.

Switch from unhealthy oils to extra virgin or virgin olive oils. Use them in place of butter. Add healthy proteins to your diet. Fish such as salmon is very beneficial. It has omega-3 fatty acids which benefits blood pressure, blood cholesterol, blood clotting and the skin. It also enhances mood and immunity. Limit red meat consumption. Also add fresh natural nuts such as almonds and walnuts to your diet.

Limit salt to less than one teaspoonful per day. If you eat generous portions of foods with high glycemic index such as baked potatoes, white rice and white spaghetti, alternative foods are suggested above along with some recipes. These would help to decrease weight as well as diseases. Adding plain low-fat or non-fat yogurt to your foods can help you to lose weight in the long run. Choose plain yogurts with limited number of ingredients. Avoid artificial ingredients.

Chapter Six

Eating Healthy Foods Including Fruits and Vegetables

Food plays a big role in our health. No one can maintain good health for a long period of time while eating the wrong foods. This is because the functions and maintenance of the body are affected by the foods that we eat. The right foods supply the right nutrients that the body needs to function effectively. The wrong foods impair the functions of the body and in some cases damage blood vessels and bring diseases upon some of the organs of the body.

Fruits and Vegetables

Fruits and vegetables are important components of healthy foods. The nutrients in fruits and vegetables benefit the body in numerous ways. Replacing unhealthy foods and snacks with fruits and vegetables is a major step toward healthy living.

Serving Size of Fruits and Vegetables

The serving size of fruits is one medium fruit or one-half of a cup of fruits. For example, one medium apple or banana is one serving. One-half of a cup of vegetables is one serving. For example one-half of a cup of broccoli or celery is one serving. For green leafy vegetables such as lettuce or spinach the serving size is one cup.

Eating Generous Amounts of Fruits and Vegetables: Benefits

(1) It helps you in the maintenance of a healthy weight

(2) It helps you in the maintenance of a healthy body

(3) It actually enables your skin to look fresh

(4) It helps you to look younger

(5) It helps you in the maintenance of healthier vision long-term

(6) It enhances your satiation and keeps you from overindulging in carbohydrates.

(7) Its generous fiber content keeps you less constipated and facilitates waste elimination

(8) The fiber also helps you to feel full so that you are not always hungry

(9) It helps regulate your bowl movement

(10)   It helps you in the maintenance of better digestive health

(11)   Juicy fruits such as cantaloupe help you keep hydrated especially in the summer

(12)   It helps decrease the space for high fat foods which can increase your cholesterol

(13)   It helps in lowering your blood pressure

(14)   Fruits and vegetables consumption help in decreasing heart attack chances, as well as stroke

(15)   The antioxidants that they contain help rid the body of toxins

(16)   It helps in preventing diverticulitis (inflammation involving the digestive tract and most commonly found in the large intestine)

Juicing and Other Forms of Fruits and Vegetables

Fresh fruits and vegetables come the way they do naturally for a reason. People often find ways of eating them that could take away from all that they are meant to offer; if eaten naturally and in their natural state. The following represent some of the forms in which fruits and vegetables are eaten:

(1) Juicing

(2) Dried fruits

(3) Canned fruits and vegetables

Juicing

If the term juicing is used to refer to the process of obtaining fresh juice from fresh fruits and vegetables, that will be a good way to get fresh 100% natural juices. This will be the case, especially, if the juices made in this way are consumed as soon as they are made and not left to deteriorate.

Blending fruits and vegetables into juice as a way of accounting for eating fruits and vegetables is a different matter altogether. The good thing about this is that it allows one to obtain available nutrients from these foods. A major disadvantage of eating fruits and vegetables in the form of juice, however, is that it denies someone the opportunity of chewing these foods. Chewing fruits and vegetables has a unique advantage. The chewing process enhances a feeling of fullness and allows someone to eat less thereby enhancing weight loss. Some people will end up eating much more food or overeating if they eat their fruits and vegetables as juice. This will cause them to gain more weight than they would have done if they chewed their foods.

If you have a medical condition that will make you unable to chew, then making juice out of your fruits and vegetables will be an excellent way of obtaining nutrients from them. Also if you have a temporal situation that requires your foods to be eaten in liquid form, making your fruits and vegetables into juice will be helpful. Some people have been unable to accommodate the eating of adequate fruits and vegetables due to extremely demanding work schedule. These people can meet this need through juicing until they are able to eat sufficient amount of fruits and vegetables. Juicing should not be the primary means of obtaining nutrients from fruits and vegetables on a daily basis.

Dried Fruits

Some of the fruits are dried before they are stored or packaged. This drying process allows the fruits to last longer. If this is the only fruit available to someone, it will be better than having no fruits at all. A major disadvantage of this process is that some beneficial nutrients are lost when the fruit is dried (including vitamins). Some dried fruits are extremely sugary.

Canned Fruits and Vegetables

Eating canned fruits and vegetables (especially those canned with water) is better than eating no fruits and vegetables at all. I will, however, not recommend canned fruits and vegetables if you have access to fresh fruits and vegetables. The healthiest diet is a diet that contains fresh and natural fruits and vegetables with no additives.

Longer Lasting Fruits and Vegetables for Busy People

Some people tend to suspend the eating of fruits and vegetables because of a very demanding schedule. If you are very busy and your fruits and vegetables tend to spoil before you can eat them, do not give up on fruits and vegetables altogether. Your good health can depend on the nutrients that they supply. Furthermore, deficiency of the nutrients that they supply can cause you to be sick and end up losing time. You can also lose a chance to maintain good weight through fruits and vegetable consumption.

The stress and expense of spoiling fruits and vegetables as well as the possibility of visitation by fruit flies can be avoided. This can be done by buying and stocking up on long lasting fruits and vegetables. Buy enough of them for one week and repurchase them each week. You can buy the others when you are able to eat them within a day or two of their purchase.

Some fruits when purchased fresh can last through most days of the week. These fruits include grapefruits, oranges, lemons, limes, apples, pears, kiwi fruit, cherries, grapes, plums, cucumber and tomatoes. I will discuss listing cucumbers and tomatoes as fruits later. Also vegetables such as broccoli, carrots and celery can last through most days of the week. This will be very good for young people especially college students, young graduates and young professionals who do not have access to fresh fruits buffet daily.

What Is the Best Thing to Eat First in the Morning?

It is best to eat fruits as the first food of the day followed by the rest of the recommended food items and vegetables. This is beneficial in a number of ways. Consuming fruits first will enhance a smooth transition from the fast through the night to the day's meals. Portion control is made easier by eating fruits and vegetables. If you need to lose a lot of weight you can drink a couple of glasses of ice cold water before your fruits.

When you eat fruits as the first food of the day avoid eating acidic fruits first. Citrus fruits are acidic; they are beneficial and are rich in vitamin C but do not eat them as the first fruit of the day. Eat them after some of the other fruits have been eaten. This is because they are among the foods that can cause heart burn when eaten on an empty stomach. Another acidic food that can cause acid reflux on empty stomach is tomato.

Consuming Adequate Fruits and Vegetables: Is It possible?

I have heard people say that it is impossible to consume the daily required number of servings of fruits and vegetables. The people who think this way fall into two groups:

(a) The first group includes those who opt for vitamin supplement to help them obtain their daily vitamins and minerals. I will discuss taking vitamin supplements in Chapter Eleven.

(b) While the second group includes those who take fruits and vegetables, not even every day but, whenever they can.

I conducted a pilot survey in July 2012 of 100 people to determine if they eat sufficient amount of fruits and vegetables daily. I chose a setting that allowed me to talk with people from different parts of the United States

On the average, only 37 % of the people I spoke to said that they eat the minimum amount encouraged per day (five servings). Of the 37 %, 8 % said that they started eating adequate amount of fruits and vegetables following an adverse event such as heart attack. They admitted noticing a significant difference in their health not long after they started eating more fruits and vegetables, avoiding sodas and making other lifestyle modifications such as exercise.

Among the people I talked with, 63 % said that they do not eat up to five servings of fruits and vegetables every day. Some of these people told me without reservation that no one can eat up to five servings of fruits and vegetables every day. I asked them if they will try from that day forward to eat more fruits and vegetables. They still said that they will do that only when they can. I mentioned to them, however, that increasing intake of fruits and vegetables beyond the five servings in a day will benefit their heart health. This will in turn help to decrease the chance of a heart attack especially if they are able to eat more vegetables. This information seemed to have convinced all but one lady that it was worth making the efforts to eat more fruits and vegetables. The lady told me that she keeps up with reading on health but is still not convinced that she could make the changes.

It is not only possible to consume the daily required amount of fruits and vegetables but it is easy to do so in spite of what some people think. You, however, have to plan for it.

Eating Enough Fruits and Vegetables Daily: The Plan

From this pilot survey, it seems that a high percentage of people eat very limited amount of fruits and vegetables daily. Some people eat a banana a day, for instance, to represent daily fruits and some carrots to account for daily vegetable intake. This could be a starting point that needs a major boost. While some people need a minor adjustment to obtain adequate fruits and vegetables, others need a radical change to accommodate adequate fruits and vegetables in their daily diet.

Make an allowance to enable you to consume sufficient amount of fruits and vegetables. Include fruits and vegetables in your foods daily in a number of ways. Be creative. When you increase the opportunities that allow you to eat generous amount of fruits and vegetables your chance of obtaining important nutrients will be enhanced. I will discuss the plan for including adequate fruits and vegetables in your daily foods. I call it the 'F.A.V.O. I.T. Plan.'

F.A.V.O I.T. Plan

What is F.A.V.O. I.T? Let us see what F.A.V.O. I.T. stands for.

F.A.V.O I.T stands for;

F-Fruits

A-And

V-Vegetables

O-On-board

I-In

T-Twos

For daily quantities of fruits and vegetables all you have to remember is the F.A.V.O I.T. Plan. It is not a diet at all. It is an uncomplicated way for you to start eating fruits and vegetables in the right way. Set a goal every week to eat a variety of fruits and vegetables by dinner time.

F.A.V.O. I.T. Plan: Including Some Examples

When the calorie intake is up to 2,000, then 10 to 12 servings (or five to six cups) of fruits and vegetables are encouraged per day. You can eat and even exceed the daily recommended number of servings of fruit and vegetables which is my recommendation and preference. This plan makes eating adequate fruits and vegetables easy, consistent, and uncomplicated.

Instead of grabbing one fruit or vegetable to represent your daily consumption of these foods, think differently. Think of the plan: when using this plan simply think of twos. Think of fruits and vegetables as if they go in twos or in pairs or as multiple servings each time. Think of reaching for your fruits the same way you think of reaching for your gloves. To help meet the hand protection goal of wearing gloves you reach for and wear them in pairs. To meet the health protective goal of fruits and vegetables it is best to reach for them in pairs or twos each time.

You should also eat each time, two servings of fruits (two fruits such as a banana and an apple) and two servings of vegetables (such as carrots and celery). This will be facilitated by having a good supply of fruits and vegetables.

I will clarify a misconception before listing the fruits and vegetables. Some people ask the question, "Are tomatoes and cucumbers fruits or vegetables?" Some fruits are usually served with vegetables in a salad, however botanically they are fruits. Botanical definition portrays fruit as a structure that bears or contains seeds. These fruits include tomatoes and cucumbers. I will list them with fruits.

Make available every week for your consumption fruits and vegetables including the following:

Fruits

Fresh apples

Fresh avocados

Fresh bananas

Fresh blueberries

Fresh cantaloupe

Fresh cherries

Fresh cucumbers

Fresh grapes

Fresh pink grapefruits (unless you take medications that are adversely affected by grape fruits even after separating medication intake and grapefruit intake by 4 hours)

Fresh kiwi fruits

Fresh mango fruits

Fresh oranges

Fresh nectarines

Fresh peaches

Fresh red, green and yellow sweet peppers

Fresh pineapple

Fresh plums

Fresh strawberries

Fresh tomatoes (including cherry tomatoes)

Fresh watermelon

Vegetables

Fresh broccoli

Fresh baby carrots (serving size 3 ounces)

Cauliflower

Fresh Romaine lettuce

Fresh onions (green, white and purple onions)

Spinach

Follow the "7 for 7 Strategy for Fruit and Vegetable Colors"

What is this "7 For 7 Strategy for fruit and vegetable colors?" This is what I call a strategy for varying the colors of fruits and vegetables that you eat daily. It will guarantee diversity in the colors of your fruits and vegetables. This will in turn maximize your chance of benefits, including the boosting of your immune system because these deep colored fruits and vegetables are rich in various nutrients.

To follow this strategy, eat fruits and vegetables representing 7 different colors and eat them 7 days a week. This will be 7 colors 7 days a week. You can eat in one day vegetables representing three different colors such as deep orange carrots, deep purple cabbage, deep green vegetables such as broccoli and spinach. You can eat fruits representing four different colors such as blueberries, yellow bananas, red grapes and pink grapefruit. These will account for 7 colors of fruits and vegetables; red, orange, yellow, green, blue, purple and pink; (ROBYGPuPi). You can add other colors some of the time such as black for blackberries.

These two ways of eating fruits and vegetables (F.A.V.O. IT Plan and 7 For 7 Strategy) remove the guesswork out of eating a variety of these foods in the right amount. It also ensures maximum benefit.

List by Color of Fruits and Vegetables for 7 for 7 Strategies: Rainbow

Red Fruits and Vegetables

Red fruits include:

Cherries

Red apples

 Hot red chili pepper

Red grapes

Red pears

Red guava

Red African mango

Red papaya

 Red sweet pepper

Pomegranate

Raspberries

Strawberries

Tomatoes

Red vegetables include

Beets

Orange Fruits and Vegetables

Orange fruits include:

Apricot

Cantaloupe

Orange African Mango

Oranges

Peaches

Pumpkin

Tangerines

Orange vegetables include:

Carrots

Blue Fruits

Blue fruits include:

 Blueberries

Black Fruits

Black fruits include:

Blackberries

Black grapes

Yellow Fruits and Vegetables

Yellow fruits include:

Banana

Lemon

Yellow sweet pepper

Pineapple

Yellow vegetables include:

Plantain

Green Fruits and Vegetables

Green fruits include:

Green apples

Avocados

Cucumbers

Green grapes

Kiwi fruit

Lime

Okra

Pear

Sweet green pepper

Green vegetables include:

Asparagus

Broccoli

Brussels sprouts

Celery

Romaine lettuce

Green onions

Spinach

Purple Fruits and Vegetables

Purple fruits include:

Figs

Purple grapes

Plums

Purple vegetables include:

Purple cabbage

Eggplant

Purple onion

Pink Fruits

Pink fruits include:

 Grapefruit

A Noteworthy Vegetable: Broccoli

Broccoli is a vegetable that is worthy of recognition. You can actually call broccoli a nutrient power house. Yeah, it may not be the best smelling vegetable but it is truly good for you. It is low in calorie. It is packed with nutrient. It is also packed with antioxidants. It contains most of the vitamins. It contains vitamin A, some of the B vitamins, vitamin C, vitamin E and vitamin K. It contains calcium and iron. It also contains fiber. It is considered beneficial against some cancers. Broccoli can be cooked or eaten raw. When eaten raw, it will retain all of its vitamins.

Cauliflower

Cauliflower is similar to broccoli in some ways. It is low in calorie. It also contains some nutrients. It contains some B vitamins, vitamins C and K. It also contains some minerals including calcium and iron. It contains some fiber. It is considered beneficial against certain cancers. It can be eaten raw or cooked. When eaten raw, it retains its vitamins.

Other food types to be made available with the listed fruits and vegetables each week include;

Gilled Fungi

Mushrooms

Mushrooms

Mushrooms are sometimes grouped with vegetables but they are actually gilled fungi. Mushrooms can be very tasty. They have some health benefits. There are edible and poisonous mushrooms. Do not pick and eat your own mushrooms unless you have expertise on mushroom recognition. Edible mushrooms are available at your local groceries. Ensure that you purchase fresh mushrooms. Fresh mushrooms have bright colors and look firm instead of shriveled. There are various types of mushrooms. Mushrooms examples include:

(a) The Agaricus mushrooms (white button mushrooms).They are commonly consumed in the United States and are believed to be immune boosting as well as cancer fighting.

(b) The shiitake mushrooms. These mushrooms have been used medicinally for centuries by Chinese and Japanese people for colds and other ailments. They seem to boosts the immune system.

Action Summary # 6

Endeavor to eat the right foods because this is very important for good health. It enhances various functions of the body that help us to maintain a healthy body and good weight. The right food supplies the body with the right nutrients. Avoid eating deceptions. There is a deception in eating that is embraced by certain people. They believe that whatever you eat should be eaten in moderation. This idea sounds good and yet it can be inadequate and misleading with regards to healthy eating. As far as food is concerned, there are right and wrong food choices. It is critical to avoid the wrong food even if it is eaten in moderation. Eat the right foods and avoid ill health over time. Good health and good weight requires commitment to healthy food choices.

Befriend your fruits and vegetables. Eat them generously everyday and they will greatly reward you. They provide various nutrients which facilitate the functions of the body. The benefits of eating fruits and vegetables include; better vision, better digestive health, better weight, enhanced elimination of toxins from the body and a host of others. Start your morning in a beneficial way as far as food is concerned. The best thing to eat first in the morning is fruits. This will allow a smooth transition from the fast through the night to the resumption of digestion in the morning. Some fruits should not be eaten on an empty stomach because they are acidic and can cause some discomfort. Eat them after the non-acidic fruits as they are also very beneficial. Examples of acidic fruits include the citrus fruits. Citrus fruits include oranges, lemons and grapefruits. Tomatoes are also acidic. If you need to lose weight, you can drink some water before your fruits.

Eat the daily required amount of fruits and vegetables and in the right way using the F.A.V.O. I.T. Plan. (See the F.A.V.O. I.T. Plan above). This plan allows you to eat the fruits and vegetables in twos throughout the day. At the end of the day with this plan your fruit and vegetable consumption will meet the daily required amount. Follow the 7 For 7 strategy to make sure that various colors of fruits and vegetables are represented in your daily foods for maximum health benefit. It is beneficial to include mushrooms in your diet. They are believed to have health benefits and decrease cancer. Broccoli is a very important vegetable to include in your diet for daily consumption. It has numerous vitamins, minerals including calcium and iron. It also has antioxidants.

Chapter Seven

Fruits, Vegetables, and Healthy Meals: Suggestions/Recipes

Some people eat vegetables soaked in additives that are very unhealthy. They contain generous amounts of fat, cholesterol and sodium and over time can do more harm than good. There are alternative ways to season the vegetables that support good health. Unhealthy dips for fruits are also problematic for health.

Seven Ways to Get the Most from Your Fruits and Vegetables

Seven Ways to Get the Most from Your Fruits

(1) Eat fruits fresh

(2) Eat them without additives

(3) Eat them with their fibers

(4) Eat them generously daily

(5) Enjoy deeply colored ones daily to maximize nutrients and benefits

(6) Ear citrus fruits such as oranges, grapefruit and lemon but not on an empty stomach as they are acidic

(7) Eat them clean

Seven Ways to Get the Most from Your Vegetables

(1) Eat fresh vegetables

(2) Eat them with their fiber

(3) Eat them with their deep color and not overcooked

(4) Eat deeply colored vegetables to maximize nutrient

(5) Eat them generously daily

(6) Eat several of them raw daily

(7) Eat them clean

Buying or Not Buying Organic Fruits and Vegetables

Organic fruits and vegetables are recommended because some non organic fruits and vegetables contain a lot of pesticides. The most important thing to consider when deciding whether or not to buy organic is whether the fruit or vegetable has an outer layer that is usually peeled off before it is eaten. The one with an outer layer that is removed before consumption has better protection from pesticides than the one that is eaten directly after washing.

Examples of fruits and vegetables that do not have to be organic include:

(1) Avocados

(2) Bananas

(3) Cantaloupes

(4) Grapefruits

(5) Kiwi fruits

(6) Lemons

(7) Limes

(8) Onions

(9) Oranges

(10)   Pineapples

(11)   Watermelons

Examples of fruits and vegetables that need to be organic include:

(1) Apples

(2) Celery

(3) Cherries

(4) Grapes (Usually imported)

(5) Lettuce

(6) Nectarines

(7) Sweet peppers

(8) Peaches

(9) Pears

(10) Plumes

(11) Potatoes

(12) Spinach

(13) Strawberries

Washing Fruits and Vegetables

Buy organic for suggested fruits and vegetables listed above as much as possible. Some people are unable to afford organic foods because of their prices. If you are unable to afford organic fruits and vegetables regularly, buy them on sale as often as you can. Some of the organic apples have very good taste and last over a week. When you buy non-organic fruits and vegetables, wash them as thoroughly as you can. You can wash them under running water with mild manual dish liquid soap diluted to one-half strength. Use kitchen towel soaked in water to scrub them (after washing with soap) to remove soap residue. Rinse them thoroughly after washing.

Scrub polished fruits, such as apples and cucumbers, carefully. Place diluted soap directly on wet kitchen disposable towels and scrub off the coating from the fruits and vegetables as much as you can. Scrub them further with clean disposable kitchen towels soaked in water. Rinse the fruits or vegetables thoroughly with water. You can also use a clean dish scrubbing brush with diluted soap to scrub the fruits and vegetables. Rinse them thoroughly with water. If you have difficulty determining whether the coating is removed from the fruits or vegetables, then wash them the day before they are needed. Observe them the next day to see if any more coating reappeared after washing. Then scrub any remaining residue off with the brush and rinse well.

For fresh green leafy vegetables, wash and rinse them individually. Sometimes some of the leafy vegetables have either some dirt or living bug sandwiched between the leaves of the vegetables. When you wash them individually you will be able to get the leafy vegetables clean and clear of dirt and bugs. Soaking them in water is discouraged.

Healthy Recipes for Vegetables

Vegetables can be eaten in a number of ways. A lot of them can be eaten raw. They can be baked, boiled, steamed and cooked in the microwave. Eating the vegetables raw supplies the most nutrient as all the vitamins are retained. Steaming for a short time limits nutrient loss. Cooking the vegetables in the microwave for less than five minutes minimizes nutrient loss.

If you are soaking in water, boiling or baking your vegetables, you may lose some nutrients including vitamins such as vitamins B and C. If you choose to boil or bake your vegetables, replace the nutrients and vitamins that may be lost. You can eat citrus fruits to supply vitamin C and nuts, raw leafy green vegetables, carrots, and fruits such as bananas and berries to supply other nutrients including the B vitamins.

Raw Mixed Vegetables

Wash, cut, and mix together the vegetables; broccoli, cauliflower, and carrots. Add to these sweet cherry tomatoes as well as red and yellow sweet peppers. You can also add some sliced mushrooms, purple grapes, and some pieces of almonds or walnuts. Serve as a nutrient rich side dish. Avoid eating these with an unhealthy salad dressing. Instead of unhealthy dressing make your own dressing. You can mix to taste some freshly squeezed lemon diluted to one-half strength with water (having the same amount of water as freshly squeezed lemon juice). Add black pepper to your taste and add olive oil. Limit olive oil to about one-half teaspoonful per person. You can be creative with making your own healthy salad dressing.

Recipe for Broccolis (Broccolis that You Can Love)

Broccolis can have good taste if they are well seasoned. Some of the seasonings have added benefits. Curry, for instance, is believed to enhance the relief of pain and inflammation. You can prepare broccolis with your favorite healthy recipe or prepare them using the following ingredients:

- 3 cups of broccoli (cut up or with branches separated)
- 3 teaspoonfuls of seasoned salt
- 2 cups of water
- 1 teaspoonful of basil leaves
- 1 teaspoonful of garlic powder
- ½ teaspoonful of black pepper
- ½ teaspoonful of nutmeg
- ½ teaspoonful of curry powder
- 2 teaspoonfuls of fresh squeezed lemon

Place the water in a deep pot and add each of the seasoning except for the fresh squeezed lemon. Stir well. Bring the water to a rapid boil. This would take about ten minutes. In the meantime, wash the broccoli and cut it up or separate the branches. Then save the broccoli in a bowl. When the seasoned water comes to a rapid boil pour in the broccoli and mix well to cover entirely the broccoli with fluid. Turn off the heat. Let stand in residual heat with the pot covered for about one minute, and then remove from heat. If you like lemon flavor pour the fresh squeezed lemon juice directly into

141

the fluid and mix well. Do not allow the lemon juice to touch the broccoli directly. The broccoli will look steamed and retain its green color. Do not overcook it. Serve them as soon as they are removed from the fluid. Discard the fluid. This will serve three to six people.

You can divide the broccoli in two. Try one half without adding lemon. Add lemon to the other half and compare the test to determine your preference. Some young people who will not touch broccoli, otherwise, love it with the lemon flavor.

The recommended daily salt intake is about one teaspoonful for people who do not have high blood pressure and less for people with high blood pressure. So it is best to discard the fluid after preparing the vegetables.

Recipe for Broccoli with Cauliflower

Ingredients:

- 2 cups of broccoli (cut up or with branches separated)
- 3 teaspoonfuls of seasoned salt
- 2 cups of water
- 1 cup of cauliflower
- 1 teaspoonful of basil leaves
- 1 teaspoonful of garlic powder
- ½ teaspoonful of black pepper
- ½ teaspoonful of nutmeg

- ½ teaspoonful of curry powder
- 2 teaspoonfuls of fresh squeezed lemon

Place the water in a deep pot and add each of the seasoning except for the fresh squeezed lemon. Bring the water to a rapid boil. This would take about ten minutes. In the meantime, wash the broccoli and cut it up or separate the branches. Also wash the cauliflower and set them aside. When the seasoned water comes to a rapid boil pour in the broccoli and cauliflower. Mix well to cover entirely the vegetables with fluid and turn off heat. Let stand in residual heat for about one minute (while the pot is covered). Remove the pot from heat. If you like lemon flavor pour the fresh squeezed lemon juice directly into the fluid and mix well. Serve them as soon as they are removed from the fluid. Discard the fluid. The broccoli will look steamed and retain its green color. Do not overcook it. This will serve three to six people.

You can set aside one-half of the broccolis and cauliflower before adding lemon. Then taste the ones with lemon and the ones without, to determine your preference. Some family members may like it with lemon.

Recipe for Mixed Vegetables I (Containing Green Beans, Sweet Red and Yellow Pepper, Carrots, Cauliflower, and Onions)

- 3 cups of the mixed vegetables
- 3 teaspoonfuls of seasoned salt
- 2 cups of water

- 1 teaspoonful of basil leaves
- 1 teaspoonful of garlic powder
- ½ teaspoonful of black pepper
- ½ teaspoonful of nutmeg
- ½ teaspoonful of curry powder
- 2 teaspoonfuls of fresh squeezed lemon

Place the water in a deep pot and add each of the seasoning except for the lemon juice. Bring the water to a rapid boil. This would take about ten minutes. Wash the mixed vegetables. Set them aside. When the seasoned water comes to a rapid boil pour them in, mix well to cover entirely the vegetables with fluid and turn off heat. Let stand in residual heat (covered) for about one minute. Remove pot from heat. If you like lemon flavor pour the lemon directly into the fluid without letting it touch the vegetables. The green beans will look steamed and retain its green color. Do not overcook them. Serve them as soon as they are removed from the fluid. Discard fluid. This will serve three to six people.

Recipe for Mixed Vegetables II (Containing Green Beans, Green Peas, Carrots and Corn)

Ingredients;

- 3 cups of the mixed vegetables
- 3 teaspoonfuls of seasoned salt
- 2 cups of water
- 1 teaspoonful of basil leaves

- 1 teaspoonful of garlic powder
- ½ teaspoonful of black pepper
- ½ teaspoonful of nutmeg
- ½ teaspoonful of curry powder

Place the water in a deep pot and add each of the seasoning. Bring the water to a rapid boil. This would take about ten minutes. In the meantime, wash the mixed vegetables. Set them aside. When the seasoned water comes to a rapid boil pour them in and stir well. Bring the water back to a boil but do not wait for a rapid boil. As soon as the water boils again turn off heat. Remove the vegetables from heat and drain. The green beans will look steamed and retain its green color. Do not overcook them. Serve them as soon as they are removed from the fluid. Discard the fluid. This will serve three to six people.

Getting It Together

Combine the above listed foods with the varied colors as much as possible. Learn to cherish various deep colored fruits and vegetables and enjoy them. With nothing to memorize, seek to obtain the daily required servings of fruits and vegetables and other foods. By the end of the day, ensure that you have exceeded the daily recommended amount of fruits. The following information is not a diet it is simply suggestions to ensure easy healthy eating every day.

Beneficial Food Groups Ratio for Vibrant Health

The amount of foods that you eat from each recommended food group is important. You can have a plan for this. A good plan can be fitted into your daily food consumption. To ensure that your eating is balanced and healthy, over three-fourths of what you eat daily should be plant based fresh unprocessed foods. Over three-fourths portions of your daily foods should be all fruits, vegetables, whole grains and some plant proteins. Allow one-half of this plant based portion to be vegetables and share the remaining half of the space between fruits, whole grain and plant proteins. This means that for every portion of whole grain that you eat you will balance it up with about four portions of fruits and vegetables with small amount of plant protein.

This will leave you with one-sixth of space left. The remaining one sixth of your daily food intake should be healthy proteins including nuts. These combine to make your full meal. You can include with the protein a glass of milk daily. You can also have yogurt. You can add fruits to salads such as sliced red or purple grapes and strawberries. Fruits should be used as desserts in addition to eating them at breakfast, lunch, and dinner.

Minimum of five to six servings per day of fruits and vegetables is considered beneficial for good health. Do not settle for the minimum amount if you want to maximize the health of your heart. Follow the ratio above and this will offer you simple easy means of eating healthy, balanced and satiating foods daily. The amount of vegetables should be more than that of fruits as this offers more benefits to the heart. Aim at about 12 to 14 servings (or six to seven cups) of fruits and vegetables every day especially if your diet has up to 2,000 calories.

A useful addition to your meals also is healthy soups with very generous amount of water. This can be part of your appetizers especially at dinner. This will help with your daily fluid intake. It will also help to increase your satiation. Eating in this way will not only allow you to obtain the nutrients that you need daily, it will also ensure that you are not hungry while eating healthy.

Suggestions for Food at Breakfast, Lunch, and Dinner

Suggestions for Food at Breakfast

It very important that you start the day with food that allows a smooth transition from the fast through the night to the resumption of digestion during the day. You can combine the various listed foods and try a different group each time. You can start your day with a variety of fruits. Use the F.A.V.O. I.T. Plan. Set a goal of two fruits (or a pair of different fruits) at a time for breakfast; one serving of each thereby broadening your nutrients from fruits. You can choose from the following fruits; avocados, small to medium bananas, cherries, grapes, grapefruit, oranges, small to medium apples (red and green). Also choose from small to medium pears, some cantaloupe (one cup), kiwi fruits, nectarines, plums, blue and black berries. You can have small to medium African mangoes two times a week. Add some celery (about one-half cup) or other vegetable to your breakfast. Also eat one boiled egg white (to supply protein) and a serving of 100% whole grain oats (oatmeal) or a serving of bran cereal. If you are concerned about gaining too much muscle, eat boiled egg whites only two to three times a week.

When you eat bread choose whole wheat bread (100% whole wheat is best) and limit number of slices to one or two. You can add low or non-fat yogurt (about four ounces) to your breakfast about three times a week, as a protein source, if you are not having yogurt for lunch. Add to your breakfast one cup of 100% natural juice. Also drink plenty of water.

You can have watermelon as well but limit quantity. It contains a lot of juice and can be very delicious. Remember, watermelon, banana and pineapples have glycemic index above 50. This means that they significantly increase the blood glucose levels when eaten. So account for that fact in the frequency of consumption and the quantity of these fruits that you consume. Eat foods with glycemic index above 49 in reduced portion. Instead of two large bananas, for instance, eat two small or two medium bananas per day. You can eat only one-fourth to one-half cup of pineapple and watermelon or include them in your meals two times a week only.

If you are looking to lose weight, eat more of the following with your breakfast daily; cherries, grapefruit and apples (choose the small apples). Cherries have low glycemic index that is less than 25, while grapefruit has glycemic index value of about 25 and apples less than 40. African mangoes have been found very useful in helping people to lose weight even though it has a glycemic index slightly above 50. You can eat one-half serving or one small mango two days a week.

About once a week or one day during the weekend you can vary your egg preparation and eat omelets. Use healthy oils such as extra virgin or virgin olive oils. Use limited egg yolk and discard the rest. When making your omelet, include only healthy items in it. You can use vegetables, including deep green vegetables and onions. You can also use deep red tomatoes, red and yellow sweet peppers, chili (hot) peppers, and mushrooms. Avoid processed meat. You can use limited amount of shrimps once a month. Clean the surfaces used for food preparation well after egg preparation.

Eggs have a lot of nutrients but it is best to eat them wisely. When you eat eggs, let it be all egg white and no yolk or egg white plus 20% (one-fifth) of the yolk for frequent consumption. This will decrease cholesterol consumption significantly. Egg yolk from two large eggs alone contain more than the daily required amount of cholesterol. Less than 300 milligrams of cholesterol is recommended daily through the diet. If you have high blood pressure, diabetes or heart disease, your daily dietary cholesterol should be less than 200 milligrams.

If you eat two large eggs with all the yolk in one day, they will supply approximately 370 milligrams of cholesterol, (about 185 milligrams per egg yolk). This significantly exceeds the daily recommended amount of cholesterol even for a healthy person. If you eat, on the other hand, 20% of egg yolk (one-fifth) per egg, you will obtain about 74 milligrams of cholesterol only from two large eggs. This minor change in egg consumption will dramatically decrease your dietary cholesterol whether you have a disease state or not. Reducing your cholesterol intake will enable you to maintain a healthier heart and keep you healthier.

Suggestions for Food at Lunch

For lunch you can eat wild caught salmon salad sandwich with no more than two slices of 100% whole wheat bread. You can use a slice of bread cut into two triangles or two slices of bread with each slice cut into two triangles. Substitute delicious low fat or non-fat yogurt of your choice for mayonnaise in the salad. You can vary your salmon salad with other salads such as vegetable salads and sandwiches. Use one-half serving size of salmon (42.5 grams) for the salad at lunch along with generous amount of vegetables.

You can add one serving of Greek or regular plain non-fat or low-fat yogurt to your lunch. The Greek yogurt has a lot of protein that will keep you full for a longer period of time. It has a lot of other benefits as well. This is very beneficial if you are trying to lose weight. Daily low-fat or non-fat yogurt consumption enhances weight loss. You can reduce the portion of your sandwich to one-half of a sandwich and add to it one serving of the yogurt. You can also reduce your yogurt size instead by choosing the four-ounce reduced portion option.

Add to your lunch nuts such as almonds. Two potions, each having six almonds per portion or 12 nuts (this is for almonds with serving size of about 24 nuts). Eat almonds about three to four days a week only, if it makes you gain weight. Eat almonds slowly by chewing one-half of a nut at a time. This will help you to eat reduced portion and also increase satiation due to prolonged chewing. You can have six almonds as appetizer and six at the end of lunch. Add two teaspoonfuls of seeds (one serving) or one-half serving to your meal as well some of the time.

Include in your lunch two different vegetables (one pair of vegetables). Choose from carrots, celery, or other. If you are eating the larger carrots, eat one carrot. You can include a small fruit in your lunch also. Choose from apples, pears, nectarines, or other fruits. Take water with your lunch instead of soda. This is critical if you want to be healthy and lose weight. Sometimes you can have a glass of 100% juice. One eight-ounce glass a day is recommended for most of the 100% juices. One-half glass or four ounces is recommended for grape juice. Drink eight ounces of green tea.

Suggestions for Food at Dinner

Include in your dinner two bowls (or cups) of different vegetables such as dark green spinach and salad with vegetables of various colors, including orange carrots, Romaine lettuce, deep green broccolis, cauliflower, and purple cabbages. Also add deep red tomatoes as well as red and yellow sweet peppers. Purple grapes (also red or black grapes) that are sliced make a really tasty addition to the salad. Avoid using unhealthy salad dressings that render the salad unhealthy. You can bake or boil sweet potatoes and add to your dinners. You can have one serving which is one medium sweet potato twice a week or one-half of a serving (about 57grams) three times a week. Adding a bowl (or a cup) of mushrooms to your dinner three to four times a week is beneficial.

Avoid processed foods and exclude them from your dinners. Add about three ounces or 85 grams of wild caught salmon (one serving) to your dinners about four to five days a week. Orange roughy (85 grams) is also a good idea some of the time. You can eat shrimp about the size of four to five jumbo shrimps or three ounces twice a week. Eat skinless poultry about twice a week and each time about three ounces or 85 grams of drumsticks, chicken breast, or thighs. Maximum frequency of poultry consumption should be three times a week.

Wash poultry thoroughly before cooking. These foods should not be undercooked. Clean the areas or surfaces where they are prepared carefully to ensure that there is no fluid left from them. Also wash your hands very well after handling them. This will minimize the chance of bacteria, such as salmonella, coming in contact with raw food like fruits and vegetables. Taking these precautions will reduce the chance of salmonella contamination. If this contamination occurs, illness (salmonellosis) will result. Symptoms of this illness include nausea, vomiting, fever, and diarrhea.

Add your favorite variety of legumes, including black-eyed peas, red kidney beans, lima beans, and lentils to your dinner menu about twice a week. Beans are healthy, high fiber, and fat free food with very low glycemic index. They, therefore, help to keep your blood glucose level low. They also help to keep your blood pressure low. They keep you fuller so you can eat less and lose weight. They are good sources of iron. They also have some calcium. Being high fiber foods, it is important to drink a lot of water with them and this can include a healthy watery appetizer soup.

For beans and peas prepare them for cooking by sorting them in large trays. Get rid of foreign bodies and damaged ones. Wash and soak them in water where needed according to package instructions. This will help the beans not to cause discomfort in form of gas or bloating. Rinse about twice before cooking in fresh water. Beans and peas can take a long time to cook so plan for that. Cooking time might be between 45 and 60 minutes. You can check them starting at 45minutes. Beans and peas are ready if they can easily be crushed.

Limit steak consumption to once a week. Maximum frequency of steak consumption should be two times a week. Eat the size of a deck of playing cards. A deck of playing cards sized steak is three ounces or 85 grams. The maximum amount of steak that you eat with your meal should not exceed six ounces or 170 grams (two decks of playing cards); and if you eat steak twice a week make the size three ounces or the size of a deck of playing cards. Eat only lean steak. Avoid frying your food. Prepare your food in healthy ways which include broiling or baking them. Avoid heavy dinners and late dinners.

 I will strongly recommend daily consumption of one-half of a large cucumber or green zucchini, raw, at dinner time or as a snack. Also make one meal of the day high fiber fruits and vegetables only. These will improve weight and health.

Customize Your Foods

You can try the different foods suggested above and combine them for breakfast lunch and dinner in the way that works best for you. Combine them also in such a way as to enable you satisfy the beneficial food ratio that we saw earlier. Also maximize nutrients; use food colors to your benefit.

If you suspect that a particular food is causing you to gain weight, skip that food for two days and note your weight for those two days to confirm whether you are gaining weight on that particular food. Isolate foods that make you gain weight and reduce their portion and frequency or replace them with an equally beneficial food. If you are gaining weight on watermelon for instance, try another fruit instead, such as pink grapefruit. Use the combinations that help you maintain a good weight. Keep your eating balanced every day. Plan your eating well so that you are not so hungry before mealtime. This is because being so hungry before mealtime can make you eat unhealthy foods. Do not stock-up on foods that you need to eat only once in a while. Buy such foods once in a while only and in small quantity and eat them sparingly.

Proximity of foods is very important. Having the right foods readily accessible helps you keep to the right foods. Make fresh fruits and vegetables readily accessible. Make wrong foods inaccessible.

Fruits and Vegetables Haters Challenge

Some people will rather eat other foods than fruits and vegetables. They do not like them. As a matter of fact, some people dislike eating fruits and vegetables as much as children dislike taking medications. I know quite a few people who do not like fruits and vegetables but consume other less healthy foods they like with predictable impairment of their health. Some people are even 'social consumers of fruits and vegetables.' This means that they eat them only when they are eating with people who encourage healthy eating. When they are alone, they quit eating fruits and vegetables.

If you do not like fruits and vegetables, regardless of your age, I encourage as well as challenge you to try many different fruits and vegetables one at a time and also in combinations. Keep trying until you find those that you like. There are numerous fruits and vegetables whose taste and health benefits will capture your attention. Try the following example:

> Make them special. Obtain a bowl that you really love. It can be a bowl that is delightfully decorated, beautifully shaped or one that has uniquely lovely prints. For a young person this can be a bowl of your favorite character. Prepare in the bowl washed, unquestionably delicious deep red, black and purple grapes. Cut up some very delicious carrots to the size of the grapes. Mix them together. Relax in your favorite spot and eat them together (one of each). When chewed together, delicious grapes and carrot pieces combine for a superior taste. This will be worthwhile as far as your health and weight are concerned. You will be improving your heart's health in the process. Your heart can thank you for it if it can speak. Even though your heart cannot thank you, your doctor's visit will have better news over time.

You can prepare any combination of fruits and vegetables that will work for you. The goal is to find out which fruits and vegetables taste good enough for you among available choices. Identifying the fruits and vegetables that you can enjoy in this way, can help to change your mind about eating fruits and vegetables. The more you like the fruits and vegetables that you have chosen, the easier it will be for you to eat them. They can boost your health and appearance if they replace unhealthy foods and snacks.

Weight Loss Foods

Sixteen Healthy Foods that Can Facilitate Weight Loss

Some foods facilitate weight loss. Some of them in spite of their fat content seem to boost the reduction of fat in the body. Add these foods to the healthy foods that you eat. You can eat one-half to one and one-half servings a day depending on the food. Vary the portion and frequency of the foods to determine what works best for you.

Foods that enhance weight loss include:

(1) Almonds (Raw and natural)
(2) Apples
(3) African mangoes
(4) Avocados

(5) Broccolis (eaten raw along with the stems)

(6) Cauliflowers (eaten raw along with the stems)

(7) Cucumbers

(8) Grapefruits

(9) Kiwi fruits

(10)   Legumes

(11)   Mushrooms

(12)   Pears

(13)   Romaine lettuce (generously green and leafy: minimum of one serving)

(14)   Salmon (choose pink wild caught salmon)

(15)   Sweet potatoes (limit it to one serving: see Baked Potato)

(16)   Yogurt: Plain, fat-free, or low-fat

Special Diet Requirement

In some situations, some people will need special diets. This happens with a lot of disease states. It can involve avoiding certain nutrients. It can also involve decreasing certain nutrients or maintaining certain balance with some nutrients. If you need a special diet, your doctor will work with you to see that you understand what is required in your new diet. In some cases you will need to work with a nutritionist to accomplish the desired goal for your health. Follow all the recommendations that you are given for better health.

Disease States and Conditions Requiring Special Diets

Medical problems that need special diets include:

(1) Congestive Heart Failure (CHF)

(2) Diabetes

(3) Food sensitivities/intolerance and allergies

(4) Hypertension or high blood pressure

(5) Kidney disease or renal failure

(6) Liver disease

Action Summary # 7

Some recipes for healthy delicious broccoli are given above. To ensure that your eating is balanced, over three fourths of what you eat daily should be plant based fresh unprocessed foods. See beneficial food group ratio above. A good goal is to aim at eating about 12 to 14 servings (or six to seven cups) of fruits and vegetables every day especially if your diet has up to 2,000 calories. Include plenty of fruits in your breakfast and eat these first. Also include 100% whole grain oats, bran cereal, boiled eggs and some vegetables. For lunch, instead of fatty hamburgers, include in your lunch salmon salad sandwiches from wild caught salmon. Also include for variety other types of salads and salad sandwiches in your lunch. Limit also the amount of bread that you use for your sandwich to no more than two slices of 100% whole wheat bread.

Add low-fat or non-fat yogurt to your lunch in addition to fruits, vegetables and some nuts. You can eat six to twelve almonds at lunch or in a day. You can have them three to four times in a week if eating them daily would make you gain weight. You can have a reduced portion option (four-ounce) of yogurt. Drink water as beverage. Sometimes you can have eight ounces of 100% juice or green tea. Avoid any soft drink or sodas.

Eat some vegetables at dinner, including dark green vegetables and salad with wide variety of colored vegetables and some fruits. Avoid unhealthy and fatty salad dressings. Add three ounces of wild caught salmon to your meals about four to five times a week and poultry about three times a week. Avoid fried food and late dinners. Adding mushrooms to your dinner is beneficial. They are delicious, and are believed to be beneficial against cancer. If your fruits tend to spoil before you could eat them due to busy schedule, buy longer lasting fruits weekly. This is a good idea for college students and young graduates also who do not have access to fruit buffet. These fruits include fresh apples, fresh grapes and citrus fruits.

Limit steak consumption to only lean steak. Also limit it to once a week or no more than three ounces twice a week. Remember that the way the cattle are fed affect the final red meat product. Cattle that are fed with grass that are not doused (drenched) with pesticides, herbicides, fungicides, and other chemicals are healthier. Cattle that are fed on grain instead of grass or exposed to various chemicals prompt health concerns.

Buy organic for the suggested fruits and vegetables that are listed in this chapter. The most important thing to consider when deciding whether or not to buy organic is; whether the fruit or vegetable has an outer layer that is peeled off before it is eaten or not. If you are not eating organic fruits and vegetables, wash your fruits and vegetables thoroughly. Ensure that polish is washed off from your polished fruits and vegetables. I listed ten foods that enhance weight loss including almonds, apples, wild caught pink salmon and lentils. Some situations make special diet necessary. These include medical problems, food sensitivities or food allergies. If you have a situation that requires a special diet, follow the diet carefully to avoid problems.

Chapter Eight

Fiber

Dietary (natural) fibers play a very important role in healthy nutrition and in good health in general. Some parts of plant that we eat are not broken down in our stomachs, neither are they digested, nor absorbed in the small intestine and they are regarded as fiber. Fiber is also known as roughage. The fiber passes relatively unchanged through the stomach, small intestine, and large intestine. It is then eliminated from the body. Large intestine is also known as the colon. Fiber, such as some cereal bran or cellulose, either pass though the large intestine without being changed or they can be partially broken down in the large intestine.

Fiber increases the amount of waste that is eliminated from the body. Daily consumption of adequate fiber enhances daily bowl movement which results in decreased waste retention by the body. Proper pharmacist counsel for patients for over the counter constipation medications includes explaining fiber facts. Fiber can be soluble or insoluble. To maximize benefit from fiber intake, it is very important to take plenty of water with the fiber.

Soluble and Insoluble Fiber

Soluble Fiber

Soluble fiber dissolves in water to form a material which is gel-like in nature. Soluble fiber slows down glucose absorption, thereby improving blood glucose levels. It can also decrease blood cholesterol levels.

Examples of soluble fibers include:

- Apples
- Blackberries
- Blueberries
- Citrus fruits
- Carrots
- Celery
- Cucumbers
- Nuts
- Oat bran
- Oatmeal
- Pears
- Seeds
- Strawberries
- Barley
- Legumes; such as beans, black-eyed peas, and lentils

Insoluble Fiber

Insoluble fibers do not dissolve in water. Insoluble fibers enhance the movement of materials through the digestive system. They will be very useful for people who are having problem with regular bowl movement. I will discuss some examples of insoluble fibers.

Examples of insoluble fibers include:

- Broccoli
- Carrots
- Celery
- Cucumbers
- Grapes
- Tomatoes
- Zucchini
- Nuts
- Seeds
- Vegetables that are leafy and dark green
- Wheat bran

Benefits of Adequate Fiber Intake

In an attempt to keep up with today's fast-paced lifestyle, many people have developed a habit of eating fast food and unhealthy snacks many of which have little or no fiber in them. These food choices which have minimal fiber content are readily available and sometimes are extremely cheap. Some people have adopted these foods and knowingly or unknowingly have deviated from daily consumption of fiber-rich foods. When less fiber is consumed, more room is left to consume foods which increase blood glucose levels and also increase body weight.

A lot of people eat less than 20 grams of fiber per day. Adequate fiber intake is about 30 grams for a 2000 calorie diet. Women need about 25 grams of fiber a day while men need about 35 grams. The goal of fiber consumption should be to meet the daily recommended amount of fiber.

Benefits of adequate fiber intake include:

(1) It decreases the risk of cardiovascular diseases

(2) It decreases the risk of type II diabetes

(3) It decreases the risk of hypertension (high blood pressure)

(4) It decreases hypercholesterolemia (high blood cholesterol levels)

(5) It decreases obesity

(6) It decreases constipation

(7) It decreases the risk of hemorrhoids

(8) It decreases the risk of diverticulitis (a painful disease which is due to the inflammation of the intestine)

(9) It help prevent overeating

(10)   It helps in stabilizing weight

Fiber and Weight Loss

Fiber plays an important role in weight loss. This is because eating a lot of fiber enhances the feeling of fullness and since the fiber will be eliminated without digestion, they could keep you full and yet not contribute to weight gain. Insoluble fibers are easily eliminated from the body. A lot of chewing goes into the eating of the fiber and since this triggers a feeling of satiation in the body, you eat less.

Fiber at Dinner

Eating a lot of fiber at dinner time is very good for you. It keeps your blood glucose level from increasing. This is beneficial for everyone. It is advantageous to diabetics who need to keep their blood glucose level low.

Recommended Sources of Fiber

Some foods when consumed on a daily basis supply adequate daily fiber. Making fiber consumption a habit can help to improve a person's overall health. Several foods rich in fiber make great snacks.

Recommended sources of fiber include:

- Oat bran
- Wheat bran
- Fresh fruits
- Fresh vegetables
- Natural nuts
- Various types of beans

It is usually a good idea to be careful what source of fiber you choose for your snack. Some people choose oat cookies for snack. Cookies belong to the group of snacks which can be chewed very fast because of their nature. As a result of this, people who choose cookies as snacks can consume a lot of calories without realizing it. It is very easy to gain weight on cookies without considering the cookies as a source of weight gain. Instead of oat cookies eat nuts, such as natural raw almonds (about 12 nuts) which has healthy fat and fiber that can help people lose weight when eaten slowly. Eating small fresh apples for snack also will allow you to gain less weight while obtaining fiber.

Fiber while promoting good health promotes good and healthy weight if successfully incorporated into the daily diet from fresh healthy and all natural sources. Avoid shortcuts when it comes to fiber. Shortcut to obtaining daily required fiber includes drinking a glass of fiber supplement.

Fiber, Constipation, and Hemorrhoids

Fiber to the Rescue

Fiber can enhance the relief of some bothersome medical conditions which are suffered daily by a lot of people. These medical conditions include constipation and hemorrhoids.

Constipation

Constipation is the inability to move the bowel with adequate frequency or having difficulty while moving the bowel. Moving the bowel at least three times a week is recommended. I will strongly recommend daily bowel movement to enhance optimal health. Constipation is a very common gastrointestinal complaint in the United States of America. The good news is that constipation in a lot of cases can be prevented.

Fiber and Constipation

Diet can play a significant role in the development or perpetuation of constipation. It is comforting to know that diet can also play an important role in the prevention or alleviation of constipation. Some people eat little fiber daily and as a result, are often constipated.

Prevention and Relief of Constipation

There are several ways to prevent or relieve constipation. The role of diet in the relief of constipation cannot be overemphasized. Movement of the bowel is regulated in the process and gastrointestinal health is maintained. Pharmacists counsel patients who want to purchase over the counter constipation medications. Proper counseling includes encouraging patients to eat high fiber diet such as fresh fruits and vegetables.

Some young children seem prone to constipation. In some cases their parents place them on stool softeners to alleviate the constipation. Some of these children avoid natural foods and so are unable to avail themselves of natural fiber that are effective against constipation. If your children are having problems with constipation, seek to alleviate it through diet. Changing what one eats is extremely effective in providing the desired outcome with constipation. This applies to people of all ages.

For everyone prone to constipation adding one serving of 100% whole grain such as old fashioned oatmeal to your daily foods is beneficial. This is in addition to eating plenty of fruits and vegetables. Specifically increase intake of both broccoli and dark green leafy vegetable, such as spinach, to two cups daily. Add to these one serving of carrots and one cup of celery daily till the constipation is resolved. Low fat or fat free yogurt eaten with fresh fruits also helps to improve digestive health. Old fashioned 100% whole grain oats (oatmeal) is a great addition to any diet whether one is constipated or not. It is worthwhile to try different possible options and determine the one that will enable you to regulate your bowel movements and avoid constipation.

Keep fully hydrated with water because inadequate fluid intake can lead to constipation. Some people have felt liberated and energized by finding relief from nagging constipation.

Additional Ways to Alleviate Constipation

Avoid sedentary lifestyle to decrease the risk of becoming constipated. Increasing your daily exercise can help with constipation relief. Add jogging and squatting exercises to your daily routine. Perform the jogging and squatting exercises morning and evening. Jog on the spot for five minutes and then follow it with the squatting exercise. Stretch your two hands out in front of you. Squat to the floor and get back up about 15 times. When you do the last squatting, hold it for 30 seconds before getting up.

Repeat the squatting exercises for five minutes. The squatting exercises along with other measures recommended will facilitate bowel movement and help to alleviate constipation.

Promptly move your bowel whenever you feel an urge for bowel movement. This is important for constipation prevention and relief. Avoid procrastination when it comes to bowel movement. Appropriate fiber intake can help you move your bowel first thing in the morning or last thing at night if that is preferred. Fiber can work in such a way as to help you move your bowel around a particular time every day. This can allow you to move your bowel at a time that is most convenient for you every day.

Hemorrhoids

Hemorrhoids are engorged (swollen) veins located in the lower rectum and anal canal. Hemorrhoids are also known as pile. Manifestations of hemorrhoids include swelling and bleeding. Internal hemorrhoids which are located in the rectal area result in painless rectal bleeding while external hemorrhoids which develop around the anal area under the skin result in severe pain in the anal area, especially during bowel movement.

Constipation and Hemorrhoids Plus Prevention

Constipation can increase the risk of developing hemorrhoids. When constipation causes straining during a bowl movement, hemorrhoids could result. I counsel patients seeking medications for hemorrhoids to avoid straining with bowel movement to help prevent or minimize hemorrhoids. Also ensuring adequate fiber and fluid intake and preventing constipation also helps to prevent hemorrhoids, which could develop as a result of constipation.

Hemorrhoids Relief

Take simple steps to obtain relief from hemorrhoids as follows:

When home remedy is indicated for hemorrhoids use ice packs or cold compresses on the hemorrhoids a few times a day; especially in the first 24 hours.

After 24 hours of cold compresses, use warm to hot water on the hemorrhoids. It is best to sit in warm to hot water for 10 to 15 minutes a few times a day. You can fill a bath tub with the water and sit in it. You can also sit in a Sitz bath filled with warm to hot water for about 15 minutes a few times a day. Sitz baths are available in your local pharmacies.

If you have limited time and are unable to sit in the bath tub or Sitz bath, you can try a quick shower option. Run warm to reasonably hot water on the hemorrhoid in a shower once a day for relief.

If your hemorrhoids do not respond to lifestyle modification and home remedies in three to four days or if it gets worse promptly consult your physician.

Minor Aches

Cold compress works very well for minor aches during the acute phase (the first 24 hours) of pain. Minor aches in various areas of the body can be addressed using hot showers after 24 hours. Before opting for medications run hot showers on aching areas such as shoulder, waist and back. As you run the shower on the area, stretch it several times. Perform some movements that cause you pain while running the hot water. Some of the body aches can be addressed profitably in this way. Do this for several days. If no relief is experienced after three days, consult your physician for evaluation.

The concept of hot and cold water compress for minor aches have been part of some cultures for generations. It dates back to ancient Egypt. It has been very successful. It sounds simple but it can be very effective. I have seen its effectiveness.

Obtaining Daily Fiber

Daily recommended amount of fiber can be eaten every day. The less processed the food you eat is, the more fiber you are likely to obtain. A lot of foods that are recommended for daily consumption contain fiber.

Examples of fiber content in some foods and snacks-are listed in increasing order of fiber content:

One cup of fresh white grapes contains about 1 grams of fiber. One cup of fresh red or black grapes contains about 1 to1.2 grams of fiber.

One small fresh tomato contains about 1.3 grams of fiber.

One medium fresh grapefruit contains about 1.7 grams of fiber.

One cup of fresh sweet cherries contains about 2 grams of fiber.

One cup of asparagus contains about 2 grams of fiber.

One serving of carrots (about 14 baby carrots or 3 ounces) contains about 2 grams of fiber, while one-half of a cup contains about 3.4 grams of fiber.

One slice of 100 % whole wheat bread contains about 2 grams of fiber, while one slice of white bread contain 0 gram of fiber.

One cup of fresh raw pineapple contains about 2.2 grams of fiber.

One medium fresh peach contains about 2.3 grams of fiber.

One cup of fresh raw sweet red peppers contains about 3 grams of fiber (while I cup of fresh raw sweet green peppers contains 2.5 grams of fiber).

One medium fresh orange contains about 3 grams of fiber.

One medium fresh banana contains about 3 grams of fiber.

One cup of cooked onion contains about 3 grams of fiber.

One serving of raw almonds (one-fourth cup) contains about 3.5 grams fiber.

One cup of fresh strawberries contains about 3.5 grams of fiber.

One cup of cooked plantain contains about 3.5 grams of fiber.

One cup of cooked brown rice contains about 3.5 grams of fiber while one cup of cooked white rice contains 0 grams of fiber.

One cup of 100 % whole grain oats (oatmeal) contains about 4 grams of fiber (serving size is one-half cup).

One cup of okra (fresh or frozen) contains about 4 grams of fiber.

One medium sweet corn on the cob or one-half cup of sweet corn kernels contains about 4 grams of fiber.

One medium fresh apple (with skin) contains about 4 .3 grams of fiber while two small fresh apples contain 6 grams of fiber.

One medium fresh pear (with skin) contains about 5.5 grams of fiber.

One medium fresh avocado contains about 5.6 grams of fiber.

One cup of cooked whole wheat spaghetti contains about 6 grams of fiber (serving size is 2 ounces or one-fourth cup).

One cup of fresh celery contains about 6 grams of fiber.

One cup of zucchini squash (raw or cooked) contains about 6 grams of fiber.

One cup of boiled broccoli contains about 7 grams of fiber.

One cup of frozen spinach (whole leaves or chopped) contains about 7 grams of fiber.

One serving (about one cup) of natural whole wheat grain and wheat bran cereal each contains about 7 grams of fiber.

One cup of cooked lima beans contains about 8 grams of fiber.

One cup of fresh red raspberries contains about 8 grams of fiber.

One cup of fresh blackberries contains about 12 grams of fiber.

One cup of cooked black beans contains about 15 grams of fiber.

One cup of sunflower seed kernels contains about 15.5 grams of fiber.

One cup of cooked lentils contains about 15.5 grams of fiber.

One cup of cooked kidney red beans has about 20 grams of fiber.

One cup of black-eyed peas contains 40 grams of fiber.

Serving Size of Beans and Peas

Different varieties of beans and peas have a serving size of one-fourth cup. When evaluating fiber content in one cup of these foods, remember to multiply the fiber in one serving by four to obtain the amount in one cup. One serving of black-eyed peas has as much as 10 grams of fiber. The serving sizes and fiber contents are indicated on the package label.

Serving Size of Nuts and Seeds

Serving size is important for the estimation of fiber content in foods and snacks. Most of the nuts and seeds have a serving size of one-fourth cup. Serving size on the package label is indicated both as the number of the nuts and the amount of nuts in one serving in a lot of cases.

Serving Size of Fruits and Vegetables

I mentioned earlier that the serving size of fruits is one medium fruit or one-half cup of fruits. The serving size of vegetables is one-half of a cup of vegetables; except for green leafy vegetables such as lettuce or spinach which is one cup.

Your Daily Fiber Calculated: Guesswork Out

Obtaining the daily recommended fiber should not be left to guesswork. The daily fiber requirement for an adult is about 30 grams. (It is slightly more for men and slightly less for women). I will discuss how the daily fiber requirement is easily met through normal healthy foods that should be in your daily diet. Examples of daily fiber in healthy foods that total up to 30 grams or more include the following;

Example one, if you eat in a day:

- One cup of fresh black grapes = about 1.2 grams of fiber
- One small fresh tomato = about 1.3 grams of fiber
- One medium fresh grapefruit = about 1.7 grams of fiber
- One cup of fresh cherries = about 2 grams of fiber
- One serving or 14 baby carrots = about 2 grams of fiber
- One cup of asparagus or one-half cup of fresh okra = about 2 grams of fiber
- One medium fresh apple = about 4.3 grams of fiber
- One cup of oatmeal (100% whole grain oats) = about 4 grams of fiber
- One medium fresh pear with skin = about 5.5 grams of fiber
- One cup of boiled broccoli = about 7 grams of fiber

Total fiber obtained = 1.2+1.3+1.7+2+2+2+4+4.3+5.5+7=31 grams of fiber

Men will need a little more fiber and women will need a little less fiber than 31 grams.

Example two, if you eat in a day:

- One small fresh tomato = about 1.3 grams of fiber

- One serving or 14 baby carrots = about 2 grams of fiber
- One medium fresh banana = about 3 grams of fiber
- One medium fresh orange = about 3 grams of fiber
- Two slices of 100 % whole wheat bread = about 4 grams of fiber
- One medium fresh red apple = about 4.3 grams of fiber
- One cup of bran cereal = about 7 grams of fiber
- One cup of boiled broccoli = about 7 grams of fiber

Total fiber obtained = 1.3+2+3+3+4+4.3+7+7= 31.6 grams of fiber

Example three, if you eat in one day;

- One cup of fresh red grapes = about 1 grams of fiber
- One medium fresh grapefruit = about 1.7 grams of fiber
- One serving or 14 baby carrots = about 2 grams of fiber
- One cup of asparagus = about 2 grams of fiber
- One medium fresh banana = about 3 grams of fiber
- One cup of oatmeal (100% whole grain oats) = about 4 grams of fiber
- One medium fresh red apple = about 4.3 grams of fiber
- One medium fresh avocado = about 5.6 grams of fiber
- One cup of boiled broccoli = about 7 grams of fiber

Total fiber obtained = 1+1.7+2+2+3+4+4.3+5.6+7=30.6 grams of fiber

Example four, if you eat in one day;

177

- One cup of fresh black grapes = about 1.2 grams of fiber.
- One small fresh tomato = about 1.3 grams of fiber
- One serving or 14 baby carrots = about 2 grams of fiber
- One medium fresh peach = about 2.3 grams of fiber
- One cup of fresh strawberries = about 3.5 grams of fiber
- One cup of zucchini squash = about 6 grams of fiber
- One cup of bran cereal = about 7 grams of fiber
- One cup of boiled broccoli = about 7 grams of fiber

Total fiber obtained =1.2+1.3+2+2.3+3.5+6+7+7 = 30.3 grams of fiber

These are just a few examples of how easy it is to keep track of the approximate amount of fiber that you are eating per day. Estimate your daily fiber intake. This does not mean that you have to get out your calculator every time that you eat. It just gives you an idea of where the foods that you eat belong in terms of fiber content. This can help you stay within a beneficial range of fiber consumption daily. If fiber is adequate in daily diet as indicated above, there will be dramatic decrease in a lot of health conditions that inadequate fiber can cause.

You only need to determine the amount of fiber that you are taking for a very limited time. You will then be able without effort to eat good amount of fiber just from choosing the right foods. This will in turn improve your health and enable you to avoid complications that can result due to ill health.

Action Summary # 8

Start today to make fiber an important part of your daily foods. Fibers play a very important role in healthy nutrition. Soluble fibers such as those from apples, citrus fruits, pears, oatmeal, beans and nuts improve blood glucose levels and decrease blood cholesterol. Insoluble fibers such as those in carrots, celery, cucumbers, tomatoes and nuts enhance the movement of materials though the digestive system and regulate bowel movement. Determine the foods that help you to maintain good digestive health including dairy products. Maintenance of good digestive health results in adequate bowel movement.

Benefits of adequate daily fiber intake include: decreased risk of cardiovascular disease, decreased obesity risk, decreased risk of Type II diabetes, decreased risk of hemorrhoids and diverticulitis. Fiber decreases blood pressure. It also improves satiation.

Avoid straining during a bowel movement. Straining due to constipation during bowel movements can cause the development of hemorrhoids. Fiber helps to alleviate constipation and so decrease the chance of developing hemorrhoids. There are also additional ways to alleviate constipation and hemorrhoids including the use of exercise. I have included a specific jog and squat exercise that is beneficial for the relief of constipation. I have included home remedies for hemorrhoids relief for anytime that home remedy is indicated.

Be aware of the amount of fiber that you consume each day by looking at the fiber values of various foods that is provided. I have included some really simple calculations that will help you to estimate your fiber intake from the foods that you can eat daily. The estimation of your fiber intake will only be necessary for a short time. You will then be able to eat the right amount of fiber by choosing the right foods. It cannot be overemphasized that you take plenty of water with the fiber.

Chapter Nine

Keep Moving

Sedentary lifestyle is an invitation for trouble as far as your health is concerned. The human body does not perform well without the benefits of good amount of movement or exercise. Incorporating exercise into your daily schedule is a major step toward good health. Regular exercise decreases the risk of a lot of diseases and problems. In counseling patients about certain medications, (such as those used for hypertension, high cholesterol and diabetes) I encourage them to exercise regularly to maximize the health benefit.

Chidi, who has expertise in fitness, clarified a lot of basic information on exercise and fitness. Exercise is a physical activity that is structured, purposeful and sustained, lasting at least 10 to 15 minutes. I have participated in extensive exercise routines, ranging from dance to limited weight training both at the gym and at home with and without an instructor.

Exercising 30 to 45 minutes at least three to four days a week is considered beneficial in maintaining good health. This is especially true if the chosen exercise increases the supply of oxygen to the lungs. Walking for a few minutes from the parking lot to an activity is better than not walking at all, but it will not constitute sufficient exercise. Consistency is the key to reaping health benefits from it.

Benefits of Physical Activities or Exercise

(1) It lowers the risk of stroke

(2) It lowers the risk of heart disease

(3) It lowers the risk of high blood pressure

(4) It lowers the risk of diabetes

(5) It lowers the risk of osteoporosis

(6) It lowers the risk of obesity

(7) It enhances bowel motility

(8) It enhances constipation relief

(9) It decreases stress

(10)   It decreases anxiety

(11)   It enhances the delivery of oxygen to the tissues

(12)   It increases energy

(13)   It helps you sleep better

(14)   It allows you to be agile

(15)   It keeps you youthful

(16)   It increases HDL (Good cholesterol)

(17)   It improves sagging skin

(18)   It enhances the removal of toxins from the body

(19)   It boosts self esteem

(20)   It enables the body to release chemicals that boost the mood

(21)   It improves your overall health

Any time I stay in a hotel, I make sure that I walk up and down the stairs for at least four floors. I avoid using the elevator. My husband encourages as many people as possible to take the stairs. He gets people taking the stairs at work. We both take the stairs often in hotels. One day, when he happened to take the elevator I opted to take the stairs at the hotel to get to the fourth floor from the first floor. We arrived at the fourth floor at about the same time. So you do not even have to lose time if you take the stairs and walk safely and briskly. I use the stairs, at work, every time I have to go from one floor to another. Usually I do this several times a day.

One day I ran into a coworker from another department at work while I was taking the stairs. She told me that she already took the stairs once that week and that using the stairs one time that week will suffice till the next week. She opted for the elevator the rest of the week. I also take a long walk when I get a lunch break at work. I safely walk briskly and use stairs, at home, several times a day.

Physical Activities: Considerations

Physical Activities

No matter what you eat if you do not exercise, over time, your health can be adversely affected. The lack of exercise, sooner or later, can enhance one disease state or the other and you can manifest symptoms that go with that disease state. Lack of exercise can also take someone from having a risk factor to manifesting a disease state. Inadequate exercise, also, results in reduced energy.

Exercise is one of those things that you will not know what you are missing until you get started with it. If you start and stay consistent, you will wonder why you had not done it earlier. Completing an exercise routine can become one of the highlights of your day. It can become a guaranteed boost to your day and mood. It can become your daily stress buster as well.

The best news about incorporating physical activities into your daily life is that your body will function better as well as look better for it. The most comforting aspect of exercise is that options are numerous and choosing a suitable exercise is easy. You can exercise for free. You can exercise for a fee. You can exercise indoors and you can exercise outdoors. You can exercise alone and you can exercise with a group of people. All you need is a determination to get started with an exercise and you have a long list of activities to choose from.

Physical Activity Considerations

When choosing a physical activity or exercise consider and answer the following eight questions first:

(1) What physical activity am I healthy enough for?
(2) What is my exercise goal? (Do I need to lose weight, or strengthen my muscles, or do I need other benefits)
(3) What can I do regularly (4 to 5 times a week) without fail?
(4) Am I increasing my oxygen intake because of my exercise?
(5) Can I sweat at least some of the time with my exercise?

184

(6) Am I strengthening my bones through my exercise?

(7) Am I strengthening my muscles to burn more calories through my exercise?

(8) What physical activity is benefiting me even in the first week of starting the physical activity?

Physical Activities Options from the Home or Hotel

Physical activities options from the home or hotel Include:

(1) Walking

(2) Jogging

(3) Running

(4) Climbing Stairs

(5) Hill climbing (And mountain)

(6) Using jump-ropes

(7) Certain shores (such as manual lawn mowing, raking leaves, scrubbing, and vacuuming large areas)

(8) Abdominal crunches

(9) Bicycling

(10)   Weight Training

(11)   Dancing with a Dance Video or DVD (Digital Video Disc or Digital Versatile Disc)

(12)   Dancing With Video Game Dance Routines

(13)   Following a Video or DVD workout routine

(14)   Aerobic exercises

(15)   Gym membership

Exercising Safely

Enjoying long term benefit from physical activity requires that you avoid exercise related injuries. Determine with the help of your physician the exercise that you are healthy enough to do. The author of this book and the publishers wish you safe exercising. They, however, will not be legally responsible for any exercise related injuries or any injuries from the use or misuse of exercise suggestions in this book. Do only those exercises that have been pre-determined to be safe for you. Some patients mention that they are unable to perform certain exercise routines. There are so many exercises that are beneficial and so it is unnecessary to participate in any one that will be inappropriate for your health condition.

Ngozi, who has expertise in health, wellness, and fitness, clarified exercise safety basics. A warm-up activity prior to exercise is beneficial. Warm-ups prepare the body for exercise. It increases blood flow. It also increases body temperature. It is helpful in preventing injury. It can involve the moves for the exercise, performed at a very low pace for a little while. For cool-downs, the moves are also performed at a very low pace for some time instead of stopping the exercise abruptly. Cooling down after an exercise helps to reduce the temperature of the muscles. It also helps to reduce injury to the muscles and also soreness that can occur after an exercise. If you are working with an instructor or a trainer, they will guide you through appropriate warm-up and cool-down moves that are suitable for your exercise. I have found cooling down from exercise so beneficial. I actually enjoy it. Wear appropriate shoes for your activities.

Do not overindulge in the activity of your choice to the point of injury. Make sure that you always have water available to you when you exercise. This is critical if your exercise is vigorous and will make you sweat. It is also very important if you are going to be hot and sweat from the heat. Some medical emergencies have resulted for some young people who were not adequately hydrated while doing sports.

Walking

When you walk for your exercise, walk briskly instead of slowly. Walking briskly or fast, which is basically walking about three and one-half miles in an hour, is more beneficial than normal walking.

Walking in Special Situations to Ward Off Sickness

I know people who have had some problems with sitting for a long time for trips. I have seen them encounter problems that range from leg swelling to varicose vein development. Simply walking, sometimes, can help to prevent certain problems.

Situations where walking can make a difference include:

(1) Long flight
(2) Long distance or cross country driving

Long Flight and Walking

When travelling on long flights, seize every opportunity to walk around and enhance circulation. This will help prevent leg swelling. Whenever possible, also, walk briskly to the baggage claim at the end of the trip instead of getting a ride to the baggage claim area. This can be a very good exercise after sitting for a long time, especially, if you are unable to incorporate exercise into your schedule for that day.

Long Distance or Cross Country Driving and Walking

When driving a very long distance, plan to stop and stretch your legs by walking. It is well worth it as this will help enhance circulation. When circulation is impaired certain conditions can manifest such as varicose veins. This is especially important for people who are predisposed to varicose veins.

Jogging

Jogging is a simple physical activity that you can use to your advantage. You can jog around your home and neighborhood. You can also jog in a scenic area such as a park or along a beach. Jogging will increase your oxygen intake which is very beneficial.

Running

You can engage in a physical activity such as running. You can run in a scenic park or along a beach. You can even run in the fields of a local high school when it is free. Running will boost your energy.

Climbing Stairs

There are so many opportunities for climbing stairs today. You can climb stairs at a local football stadium, at work, or at a hotel. You can even climb stairs at a local mall. You can climb the stairs safely and briskly. Climbing stairs can be a very simple and profitable way to stay active.

Hill Climbing (And Mountain)

Hill climbing is a beneficial way to stay active. I will emphasize carrying some water with you for hill and mountain climbing. A personal trainer can help to prepare you for climbing the hill and mountain.

Exercising with Jump-Ropes

Jump-ropes are easy to store and carry around. Using jump-ropes can be a great way to exercise. You can use the jump-rope in your house, in a scenic park, or on a beach. Jumping rope tones several muscles in the body including the muscles in the arms and legs. It benefits the whole body. You can rest by walking a few steps or for one minute and then continue. Jumping ropes can be a great fun exercise for kids as well.

Abdominal Crunches

Abdominal crunches are part of the core exercises that help strengthen your core muscles. You can do it on a portable exercise mat. This is a good exercise to help you prepare for riding a bicycle. When your stomach muscles are strengthened and your stomach flattened, your health will be enhanced; since belly fat is associated with a number of diseases.

Certain Household Shores

Certain household shores can serve as exercise sometimes. These household shores include manual lawn mowing, raking leaves, scrubbing, and vacuuming large areas. Do not rely on household shores alone for your exercise. Supplement your household shores with additional exercises that will increase your oxygen intake.

Bicycling

Bicycling can be a good exercise. You can ride your bicycle around your neighborhood or along a scenic route. Carrying water along with you on your bike rides is very important.

Weight Training

Check with your doctor before lifting weights. Make safety a priority in weightlifting. You can get help with a fitness expert such as a fitness trainer in the beginning if necessary; until you are comfortable. Lift only the weights that your body can handle. Weights training can be performed using free weights such as dumbbells and barbells or weight machines. Weight lifting has benefits that include; fat reduction, strengthening of the bones, enhancing muscular strength, and endurance. It tones abdominal and other muscles.

Sagging Skin and Weightlifting

Some people have skin that is loose or sagging. This could occur due to weight loss or aging. If you have this situation, add weight training to your weekly exercise about twice a week to help firm the skin.

Dancing with a Dance Video or DVD

Dancing with a Video or DVD can become a great modern day getaway for ladies. Ladies' get-together can be crammed with benefits if they add a 30 minute dance workout routine to it. It can be a fun activity to do together. It can also save the ladies some time since their daily exercise can be accounted for by this outing. It can also be a profitable activity for home schooling parents who are teaching teenagers. It will serve both as a social event and exercise.

Dancing with Video Game Dance Routines

Some video games have dance routines for exercise. This can be an excellent way for young children and teenagers to exercise. The whole family can even exercise together sometimes using these dance routines. They are a lot of fun and can help people to burn calories as well.

Following a Video or DVD Workout Routine

There are several workout videos and DVDs that are now available. Some of them are easy to follow and can be finished within 30 minutes. Invest only on workout routines that you are able to perform and enjoy.

Aerobic Exercises

Aerobic exercises are physical activities whose movements cause the heart and lungs to work harder as a result of increase in the demand for oxygen. Aerobic exercises cause more oxygen to be delivered to the organs and tissues. Aerobic exercises lead to sweating. Some people call aerobic exercises cardio workout.

Aerobic exercises include; running, cycling, swimming, jogging, and aerobic dance routines.

Gym Membership

When we got a gym membership for the whole family, I was impressed by all the exercise options that came with the membership. It included opportunities for swimming, dancing, treadmill, weight lifting and other activities. If your schedule allows for frequent visit to the gym, it will be one of the options that you will consider. If you are one of those people, however, who feel good about having a gym membership; and yet are unable to make it to the gym day after day, cancel the membership and save your money. You can choose one of those exercise measures that you can avail yourself of 24 hours a day.

Exercise Combinations

It is a very good idea to combine your physical activities instead of just participating in the same routine always. Combining your exercise routines is known as cross-training. You can jog or run and also perform exercises that include stretching such as Yoga. You can also jump rope and swim instead of jumping rope alone. This cross-training will help prevent overuse injury.

I observed a lot of overuse injuries sustained by some athletes who were participating in various sports. Overuse injury include bone injury such as stress fracture or muscle injury such as tendonitis. If you are concerned about injury or if you are not meeting your exercise goals, work with a personal trainer for some time to help you exercise safely and achieve your goals.

Exercising without Excuses

Sometimes you might have a very busy schedule and finding time to exercise might seem impossible. Unfortunately this can happen rather frequently with certain jobs and schedules. The best thing to do in this situation will be to follow a combination routine that is easy to do without much preparation. I call it the "excuse buster routine." Find the safest area near where you need to be or where you are working. You can even use one side of a room. You will need a pair of sneakers. Change shoes and put on appropriate pair of sneakers. If you can wear something comfortable do so if not, remove belt or tie and make what you are wearing as comfortable as possible.

Choose the side of the room that is most spacious if you are unable to go outside. Set an alarm to go off in 30 minutes with a cell phone or use a timer. You can also try two sessions each lasting 15 minutes if that fits better into your schedule. Adapt and perform three of the exercises that are considered beneficial; jumping rope, jogging, and brisk walk. One way to do this is to jump rope in this area. Ensure that you are moving your hands as if you are using a jump rope even if you do not have a jump rope with you. Walk briskly some of the time in between jumping rope. As you are walking, tuck in your stomach and release it. Repeat the tucking in and release of your stomach throughout the brisk walk. Jog also. Do this some of the time. Alternate jump rope motions with walking briskly also. Do all these moves until your alarm rings. Cool down. Following these routines will allow you to exercise in spite of a difficult and demanding schedule.

Exercise and Insomnia

Avoiding vigorous activities just before bedtime is part of good sleeping hygiene. Exercising close to bedtime can keep some people from falling asleep. It is best if you complete your exercises up to five hours before bedtime so that your sleep will not be adversely affected. The key is to complete exercise several hours before you go to bed. You may need to experiment to see what works for you. Some people need to allow more time between exercise and bedtime than others.

Former Athletes, Young Adults, Plus College Graduates and Exercise

Some athletes seem unprepared for reduced exercise or life after athletics. One of the worst things a former athlete can do is to live a sedentary lifestyle from daily vigorous exercise. This includes exercising only whenever and wherever possible. Such dramatic change in exercise and fitness could result in uncontrolled weight gain and certain disease states that are enhanced by excess weight. It will also adversely affect muscle mass especially for males. It is best to plan on continuing to exercise for life following athletics. I have seen a lot of athletes gain much weight following completion of college athletics. Some admit to being out of shape or too busy to exercise.

No dramatic routine is necessary. Just make room for any aerobic exercise for 30 to 45 minutes, about four to five days a week. If your schedule is tight, that would not be a problem. Opt for 15 minutes exercise plans, two to three times in one day.

This is not only good for former athletes. It is a great idea also for all young adults including college graduates some of whom, helplessly, watch their weight increase beyond expectation after college. Do not wait till your weight doubles before you do something about regular exercise. You do not need your schedule to get better either. Incorporate any beneficial exercise into your schedule.

Even busy moms can benefit from this as well. Also busy career persons can participate in exercise as well in this way. This allows a person to exercise regardless of their schedule. Health is boosted in the process, while at the same time adhering to a busy schedule. If a busy schedule is allowed to stop one from exercising, health could be diminished. Diminished health will end up working against your schedule by slowing you down or even stopping you from doing your work in the first place.

Seniors and Exercise

Some people may think that seniors do not have to worry about getting regular exercise. On the contrary, exercise is very important for seniors. If you are a senior adult, make exercise an important part of your week. It will enhance the health of your heart and help to strengthen your bones and muscles, as well as help to boost your moods.

Talk to your doctor before you start your exercise. There are several exercises to choose from. Dance exercises, swimming exercises and climbing stairs work very well for some seniors. Some seniors really enjoy aerobic dance. Others do weight training. Start slow and increase intensity of your exercise slowly over time. Pay attention to your body when you exercise and respond to the way your body is feeling. Do not overstretch yourself to the point of injury.

Disabled Persons and Exercise

If you are disabled, talk to your doctor before you exercise. Use the help of a fitness trainer if possible to get the benefits of exercise. There are some exercise equipments that could facilitate exercising with disability. Explore different exercise possibilities to see what would work best for you. All the hard work that you put in will indeed pay off. Exercising safely as much as you are able would give your health a boost.

Action Summary # 9

Exercise regularly and adhere to a regular routine that you are healthy enough for. Regular exercise promotes good health. Check with your doctor before you start exercising to determine carefully the exercises that are safe for you. There are various exercises to choose from. Do not allow a busy schedule to keep you from exercising thereby diminishing your health. Diminished health will end up slowing you down. When you are travelling long distances by air or by road seize every opportunity to walk. This will prevent circulation from being impaired. Former athletes should continue to exercise as well as young adults. Seniors, with their doctor's, approval should choose exercise routines that they can participate in. Persons with disabilities can exercise with the help of a fitness trainer.

It is recommended that you complete your exercise routine several hours before bedtime so that your ability to fall asleep will not be adversely affected. You may exercise five hours before bedtime. You may experiment, also, to know how many hours you need to leave between exercises and bedtime.

Chapter Ten

Obstacles to Healthy Living

Everybody wants to live a healthy and happy life. People try all kinds of things in an attempt to be healthy. There are certain problems that keep people from enjoying a healthy life and all the benefits that it offers. Sometimes, I have uncovered obstacles that patients have to healthy lifestyle during medication counseling. My health survey further revealed obstacles to good health. These include obstacles affecting emotional health.

Identifying and resolving various obstacles to healthy living can be the link between knowledge and implementation of a healthy lifestyle. I will discuss some of the obstacles that can stand in the way of a healthy lifestyle.

21 Obstacles to Healthy Living Include:

Part A

(1) Influence

(2) Environment

(3) Unhealthy habits

(4) Poor dental hygiene

(5) Insufficient sleep and poor sleeping hygiene

(6) Difficult schedules: No time for healthy foods?

(7) Procrastination

(8) Lack of accountability

(9) Desires

(10)   Meal course orders (A multi-course meal)

(11)   Large meal portion traditions

(12)   The love of sugars and candies

(13)   Financial limitations

Part B

(14)   Stress

(15)   Negative impact and negative thinking

(16)   Unforgiveness

(17)   Lack of self acceptance

(18)   Lack of confidence

(19)   Isolation

(20)   Depressed state (Discouragement)

(21)   Fear

Part A

Influence

Influence can be positive or negative. Positive influence includes encountering people that inspire you to accomplish great things in your life. Negative influence on the other hand includes encountering people who hinder your progress in your life endeavors or in your health. Some people have friends who have unhealthy habits of smoking cigarettes. As a result of the influence of their friends they pick up smoking and end up becoming regular smokers. This can eventually lead to a life threatening addiction. Some people also start drinking alcohol because of the influence of their friends. It can also start as a social obligation and end up becoming a life altering addiction.

Sometimes, the influence of friends and co-workers can encourage unhealthy eating. A lot of people have gained weight and eventually became overweight in this way. When some people eat out with friends and co-workers, they tend to choose the most delicious, least healthy entrées from the least healthy restaurants or the least healthy entrées from any restaurant menu. Some people eat out often with their friends and co-workers and over time, the unhealthy foods take their toll not only on weight but on health also. People can become less concerned about unhealthy weight if their friends have unhealthy weight as well.

Suggestions Concerning Influence

Endeavor to choose friends who will support you in your efforts towards a healthy lifestyle. Avoid friends who will make you falter in your efforts to be healthy. Socializing with friends who smoke cigarettes or drink alcohol opens you up to a chance of addiction to cigarette smoking or indulgence in alcohol; which will diminish your health.

Have an agreement that if you get together with people who have problems with smoking cigarettes or drinking alcohol, you will exclude alcohol and cigarettes from your activities throughout your time together. Do a sporting activity together instead and get your daily exercise while you are together and that will benefit every one of you. I will discuss smoking and alcohol in greater detail later.

Strive to be part of the solution rather than part of the problem. Come up with suggestions to make your meal outings healthier. You can encourage your friends and co-workers to only indulge in unhealthy foods no more than once in a month. You can all bring your own healthy foods and have lunch together. You can have weight loss competitions among your friends and co-workers monthly with prizes. Adjustments such as these can help you and your friends to avoid being overweight. This will in turn keep you and your friends healthier.

Environment

Environment can affect people's health. Some people have very easy access to foods that can diminish their health. They live or work close to convenience stores that have a variety of unhealthy foods and snacks which are often on sale. In addition, some people live or work close to some fast food restaurants. They become accustomed to eating in these restaurants on a daily basis. Over time frequent consumption of unhealthy fast foods will lead to weight gain and coronary artery disease. Also some people are surrounded by people who are negative examples and who make poor life choices.

Suggestions Concerning Environment

It is very tempting to opt for quick foods and snacks from convenience stores and fast food restaurants. Resist the temptation to rely on quick and unhealthy foods. On the contrary have a plan to prepare healthy foods for yourself every day. If you must indulge in unhealthy quick foods, do that only once in a month. Eat reduced portion of these foods. Replace unhealthy snacks with healthy ones. Some snacks such as fiber containing nuts can taste very good and can be great alternatives to unhealthy snacks.

If you are always around people who are not good examples and who make poor life choices; seek out and stay around people who are good examples and who make healthy life choices. Young people can participate in mentoring programs. Associate with people who can make you better rather than worse.

Unhealthy Habits

There are various habits that stand in the way of a healthy lifestyle. Habits can be difficult to break but a habit that impairs good health is best discontinued. If you eat foods such as doughnut, croissants, sugar cookies, and other pastries at breakfast every morning or pizzas for dinner, you will be unable to optimize your health. Pastries and pizzas are not recommended for frequent consumption.

Some people have a habit of sitting for hours in front of the television and watching whatever comes along. Most of the time this prolonged watching of the television is accompanied with snacking on things such as potato chips. Watching the television for hours is not healthy. Snacking for a long time on potato chips can lead to over indulgence on potato chips which will eventually lead to ill health.

Suggestions Concerning Unhealthy Habits

There have been some cultural allusions to the fact that you cannot change a long standing habit. Such sayings include the allusion that you cannot learn to be left handed when you are old. When it comes to your health, change can and should be made any time that it is indicated for good health. Adhering to long standing habits can potentially hurt you. If you have a habit of eating unhealthy foods, change to good healthy foods. Discontinuing unhealthy foods and snacks can be a major step towards achieving a healthy lifestyle. Healthy foods and snacks will boost your health, including your heart health. Add healthy activities to your daily schedule and discontinue activities such as watching the television for hours.

Poor Oral Hygiene

Pharmacists sometimes have to recommend oral care products to patients. Good dental health is important to me. I take good oral hygiene recommendations seriously. I have watched good oral hygiene videos. I have included basic information that will enhance good dental health in this book.

Poor oral hygiene can adversely affect your overall health. Neglecting simple habits that improve dental health can result in some dental problems such as the development of cavities or even periodontal disease. If oral bacteria are left undisturbed either on the front, back or in-between the teeth, dental plaque can form on teeth. Dental plaque is formed when free floating oral bacteria form colonies and stick to teeth. Dental plaques absorb and change sugars in food and candies. They produce acids in the process. Acids from plaques demineralise teeth, removing calcium from teeth which result in cavities. Activities from bacteria in the plaque also cause gum inflammation and bleeding. Dental plaques over time cause destruction of the gum around the teeth. This results in gingivitis; which is a form of periodontal disease. Periodontal disease results from infection and inflammation which destroy tissues around the teeth.

Symptoms of periodontal disease include;

- Swollen gum
- Reddish gum
- Bleeding gum
- Tender gum when touched or when brushing

Signs of Dental Cavities

Signs of dental cavities include;

- Holes that can eventually be seen in the teeth
- Toothache especially when something sweet, hot, or cold is eaten

If dental problems occur and give rise to toothache, productivity will decrease and health will diminish. If dental problems are not evaluated and treated tooth loss may occur.

Be Aware of and Care about Your Breath

"What has bad breath to do with health?" you may ask. Unfortunately, consistent bad breath can be an indication of poor dental health. It can also be the result of a dental disease such as tooth decay or periodontal disease. Consistent presence of excess bacteria loads in the mouth cause dental health to deteriorate. When the condition of the teeth is deteriorating due to excess bacteria load, bad breath increases.

Dental Health

What Does Stroke Have to Do with Dental Health?

Increase in oral bacteria is a consequence of poor dental health. Bacteria present on teeth and gum can enter the bloodstream. The bacteria can then become attached to fatty plaques in the arteries. The bacteria can increase inflammation of the fatty plaque. If a plaque bursts and results in clot formation, a stroke may occur. Poor dental health, therefore, can increase the chance of getting a stroke.

Suggestions Concerning Poor Oral Hygiene

Take good care of your teeth. Practice good oral hygiene daily. Take all the basic but critical steps to ensure good dental health. Add to daily brushing of your teeth daily flossing also. Brush and floss your teeth twice a day. This is very important for your dental health. Some people have brushed their teeth twice a day diligently in an attempt to maintain good dental health. They, however, omitted the flossing of their teeth. To their surprise, over time, they developed a dental problem; a cavity or periodontal problem. Brushing your teeth daily without flossing them is not enough. Flossing your teeth is an essential component of good oral hygiene. Flossing will help remove the plaque and decaying food that are stuck between teeth.

While flossing, place the floss over each tooth at the gum line and make a half moon shape. The floss should be positioned gently between the tooth and gum. Hold this against the tooth and floss. Also brush the chewing surfaces of the teeth. Good brushing and flossing will help give your dental health a boost. Clean and brush your tongue thoroughly every day while brushing your teeth. Tongue cleaning will remove the white or yellow coating of bacteria on the tongue.

Bacteria reduction in the mouth is always a good thing. Be thorough with the up and down movement of your brushing technique. Ensure that you brush vertically towards the gum, up and down daily to dislodge and ward off any developing plaque. Plaque control is very important for good dental health.

Rinse your mouth daily with a good mouthwash to kill germs. It will be very beneficial to use the mouthwash after flossing your teeth. If you do not have access to mouthwash, add iodized table salt (about 2 teaspoonfuls) to a cup of warm to relatively hot water and rinse your mouth with it until you can obtain a mouthwash. Do not swallow the salt water. Rinse your mouth thoroughly with water following the salt rinse.

Flossing the teeth and rinsing the mouth with a mouthwash after flossing will not only decrease bacteria load in the mouth; it will also help decrease bad breath. As you go through the day, try to refresh your breath with quick rinsing of your mouth with water. This will also help to reduce any food particles that bacteria can work with and cause problems in the mouth. Do this a few times a day even at work. This will help you to maintain good breath and also enhance your dental health.

If you take good care of your teeth and go for routine dental check-up, daily use of mouthwash will not be as critical. However, to minimize dental problems due to bacteria and to achieve additional protection, it is a good idea to take advantage of daily mouthwash use. Use mouthwash brands that are approved by the national dental association. Replace your toothbrush after about 4 months. These will result in healthier teeth, mouth, and body.

Consistent good breath is an indication of good oral hygiene and healthy teeth. Good oral hygiene is good for your overall health. I cannot emphasize good oral hygiene enough. My sister, Dr. Ify Nwabugwu, who is a dental surgeon and I discuss oral health sometimes.

Insufficient Sleep and Poor Sleeping Hygiene

The body needs a lot of rest to continue to function effectively. When I counsel patients who try to take over the counter sleep aids routinely, I encourage them to practice good sleeping hygiene. Getting six hours of sleep at night as minimum is barely enough for optimal health. A lot of people are unable to get sufficient sleep at night. Insufficient sleep on a consistent basis is also an obstacle to good health. Busy daily schedule might require some planning to accommodate adequate sleep. Getting adequate sleep should not be left to chance.

Good sleeping habits include actions that make falling asleep easier. Some actions or situations can keep people from either falling asleep or getting sufficient sleep at night. Problem with sleep is one of the most common complaints that make people buy over the counter medications. Pharmacist's counseling of patients seeking over the counter sleep aids involves questions regarding their health conditions and medications to identify those who need medical attention. It also entails enquiry about the duration of the sleep problem and previous treatments. Proper patient education and counseling for sleep problems include explaining to the patient good sleeping hygiene basics and their importance.

Causes of insufficient sleep or lack of sleep include;

(a) Vigorous exercise just before going to bed

(b) Stress

(c) Alcohol

(d) Stimulants such as caffeine and nicotine

(e) Change in work schedule

(f) Change in time zones

(g) Frequent late night outings

(h) Discouragement

(i) Worry

(j) Bed discomfort

Vigorous Exercise Just Before Going to Bed

Time of exercise is important with regard to sleep. Vigorous exercise close to bedtime is part of poor sleeping hygiene and this could prevent you from falling asleep. If you exercise within four hours of bedtime your sleep might be adversely affected.

Stress and Sleep

Stress can keep you from sleeping at night. If you go to bed while under a lot of stress, you might be unable to fall asleep. Your chances of getting a good night's rest will be greatly diminished.

Alcohol and Sleep

Taking alcohol and going to sleep can prevent a good night's sleep. Alcohol is a sedative. It will allow you to fall asleep but it will not allow deep sleep. It could cause an interruption in your sleep by causing you to wake up in the middle of the night and as such not be rested at night.

Stimulants and Sleep

Beverages such as tea and coffee contain caffeine. Caffeine is a stimulant which if taken in the evening can prevent you from going to sleep at night. Nicotine in tobacco is also a stimulant which can keep you from falling asleep as well.

Change in Work Schedule and Sleep, Change in Time Zones and Frequent Late Night Outings

A change in your work schedule can affect your sleep adversely. Schedules such as night shifts adversely affect the circadian rhythm of your body. The circadian rhythm directs your sleep and wake cycles. Working at night instead of sleeping for a sustained period of time disrupts this natural internal clock of the body and so affects sleep.

Travelling to different time zones also disrupts the circadian rhythm and affects sleep. This disruption of sleep patterns due to change in time zones is particularly significant for international trips where time difference between the country of origin and the destination country can be five or more hours.

Frequent late night outings can also disrupt your circadian rhythm. Disruption of your sleep and wake cycles can cause daytime fatigue. This can affect productivity during the day, eventually, if sustained.

Discouragement and Sleep

Discouragement can keep you from falling asleep at night. If you continue to reflect on your discouragement, you will be unable to get rested at night. If this continues, your health will be adversely affected.

Worry and Sleep

We all know that the act of worrying does not diminish the problem that we are concerned about and yet we worry about the problem anyway. Time spent in worrying about problems rather than resolving the problems does not contribute to relief. Some people worry until they develop chest pain or a headache both of which diminish health and add to the prevailing problems rather than offer solution to the problems.

Bed Discomfort

The condition of a bed can play a role in one's ability to fall asleep. Comfortable beds enhance sleep. Bed discomfort can adversely affect sleep.

Addressing Problems with Sleep

Some of these people who have problems with sleep place themselves on over-the-counter sleep-aids. Taking medications without addressing obstacles to sleep will only make matters worse.

Suggestions for Insufficient Sleep and Poor Sleeping Hygiene

Avoid performing vigorous exercise close to bedtime. Finish your exercise four to five hours before bedtime so that your sleep will not be adversely affected. If you cannot fit your exercise into your schedule four to five hours before bedtime, still do the exercise to enhance your health. Adjust the exercise time, however, to the time that will not significantly affect your sleep. You may have to experiment with different times. Reduce the intensity of night exercises to the level that will allow you to sleep at night. Avoid reflecting on your problems when you go to bed. You can take a book into bed and read yourself to sleep.

Even though alcohol is a sedative that can allow you to fall asleep, it is a good idea to avoid it. Do not take alcohol close to bedtime. Taking alcohol before going to sleep can prevent you from getting a good rest at night. If you go to sleep under the influence of alcohol, you might wake up in the middle of the night. Be aware of this and avoid this sleep interruption and negative effect on your sleep.

Taking stimulants could adversely affect your sleep at night. Avoid drinking beverages (such as tea or coffee) that contain caffeine late in the evening so that you will be able to fall asleep at night. Avoid the use of cigarettes close to bedtime. Nicotine in tobacco can keep you from falling asleep.

I have travelled several times and spent several weeks in places separated from my starting point by six hours. I finally put a plan together to allow for minimal jet lag upon my return. When you travel to a different country or to any place that is in a different time zone, adjust your sleep time to conform as much as possible to the place that you came from when possible. If your country of origin is five hours ahead of the country you are spending time in, for instance, then go to bed at about 9:00 pm, if possible, so that you can get some sleep before it is late morning in your country of origin. If you go to bed at 9:00 pm and wake up at about 4:00 am, for instance, you would have slept for seven hours and it would be 9:00 am in the country you came from. If you happen to sleep late, it would be mid-day or afternoon in your country of origin by the time you wake up.

Adjusting your sleep time will help to minimize the disruption of your sleep. Working a night shift is similar to being in a different time zone. When working a night shift be sure to sleep as soon as possible in the morning.

Going out late at night is a problem. Avoid frequent late night outings which can disrupt your sleep and wake cycles. When beds become uncomfortable enough that people use time meant for sleep to toss and turn in discomfort, a change of bed is worthwhile.

When you are discouraged, try to resolve as much of your issues as possible before you go bed. Talk to someone you trust for encouragement. Avoid reflecting on discouraging issues once you lie down to sleep. Distract yourself from the discouragement by reading yourself to sleep after talking to someone that you trust.

Seek help with your bothersome problems. God cares about your worries and is able to help you. 1 Peter 5:7 says "leave all your worries with Him, because He cares for you" (Good News Bible). You are asked to seek the kingdom of God and all the things we usually worry about "shall be added to you," Luke 12: 31 (New King James Version). You can also ask for prayers for your problems. Some radio and television stations even pray for people. When you go to bed, however, do not continue to worry about your problems. Lack of sleep, unfortunately, will add to your problems.

Practice good sleeping hygiene to help you sleep and get good rest. Do not resort hastily to sleep aids. Under normal circumstances, good sleeping hygiene will make a big difference in your ability to fall asleep, stay asleep, and get rested at night. If your inability to sleep is due to a medical condition that needs to be addressed first, you will need to consult your physician.

Difficult Schedules: No Time for Healthy Foods?

Limited Time to Prepare Healthy Foods

Some people have schedules that leave insufficient time for the preparation of healthy foods. I know of people who at the end of the day go home tired and very hungry. Having a limited time to prepare food, they boil generous amount of hot dogs and eat them for dinner. This type of food results in weight increase and over time will increase the risk of coronary artery disease. It can diminish health in a way that will result in lost work time and expensive medical attention.

Suggestions Concerning Difficult Schedules

Finding ways to better manage time can help tremendously when one has difficult schedules. This can involve doing things differently from what one is used to. I had no choice but to determine how to make healthy dinners on an impossible schedule. It was the only way I could complete a doctoral program, which ran only a full time schedule, and still be a mother of four children who were very busy with various sports and other activities.

Some healthy dinners can take almost the same time to prepare as unhealthy foods such as hot dogs. Prepare simple dinners that will be ready within 30 minutes. There is no need to eat heavy dinners.

Example of a Quick Healthy Dinner

You can use fresh salmon fillet with scales removed or frozen ones. If you are using frozen salmon fillet, put them in the refrigerator to defrost overnight. It might need about nine hours. You can also leave it sealed in the refrigerator till you are ready to make dinner. When you are ready to make dinner, and as soon as you wash your hands, preheat oven to 425 degrees. This could take ten minutes depending on the type of oven. Start baking about six washed salmon filets in the heated oven. You can use the recipe below.

Salmon Recipe

- 6 washed salmon fillets (24 ounces)
- 1 and ¼ teaspoonfuls of seasoned salt
- 1 teaspoonful of basil leaves
- 1 teaspoonful of garlic powder
- ¾ teaspoonful of nutmeg
- ¾ teaspoonful of curry powder
- ¾ teaspoonful of black pepper
- I and ¼ cups of fresh onions sliced into six in ring form

Place the salmon fillets in a baking pan. Sprinkle with the seasoned salt or use an empty salt shaker to sprinkle the measured salt evenly on the fish. Add basil leaves, black pepper, nutmeg, curry, and garlic powder. Spread each ingredient evenly on the salmon fillets. Then place the onion slices on the fillets (one for each fillet). Cover with a second baking pan. Avoid using aluminum foil in baking food or covering hot food. Start baking as soon as the oven is heated to 425 degrees and bake for six or seven minutes. The timed oven would then turn off. Let stand in residual heat for about four to five minutes or until the fish crumbles when poked with a fork. Remove from heat. Do not overcook or dry the salmon. The salmon dinner should be ready in less than 30 minutes. This serves about six people.

Almond Salmon Delight Recipe

- 6 washed salmon fillets (24 ounces)
- 1and ¼ teaspoonfuls of seasoned salt
- 1 teaspoonful of basil leaves
- 1 teaspoonful of garlic powder
- ¾ teaspoonful of nutmeg
- ¾ teaspoonful of curry
- ¾ teaspoonful of black pepper
- I cup of fresh onions sliced into six in ring form
- 24 crushed and partially ground almonds

Place the salmon fillets in a baking pan. Sprinkle with the seasoned salt and spread evenly on the fish or sprinkle evenly the measured salt using an empty salt shaker. Add basil leaves, black pepper, nutmeg, curry, and garlic powder. Spread each ingredient evenly on the salmon fillets. Then place the onion slices on the fillets. Place one slice on each fillet. Start baking as soon as the oven is heated to 425 degrees. Cover with a baking pan and bake for six to seven minutes. The timed oven would then turn off. Let stand in residual heat for four to five minutes. Ensure that the salmon crumble when poked with a fork, but do not overcook or allow the salmon to become dry. Sprinkle the almond on the fillets and let stand for one minute. Then remove from heat. The crushed almonds should not stay in the oven for more than one minute. The salmon should be ready in less than 30minutes. This will serve about six people.

You can eat it with raw vegetables. For raw vegetables (salad), you can wash, cut as desired, and mix together broccoli, cauliflower, carrots, red and yellow sweet peppers. Add to these sweet cherry tomatoes, cucumber and deep colored leafy vegetables. You can also add some sliced mushrooms, purple grapes, and some pieces of almonds or walnuts. Serve as a nutrient rich side dish. Avoid eating these with an unhealthy salad dressing. You can make a healthy salad dressing of your own. You can mix to taste some freshly squeezed lemon diluted to one-half strength (Add the same amount of water as freshly squeezed lemon juice). Add to your taste, black pepper and then olive oil. Limit olive oil to about one-half teaspoonful per person. Be creative with making your own healthy salad dressing.

You can also cook your vegetables. You can cook them while the salmon is baking in the oven. If you cook your vegetables replace lost nutrients which include vitamins B and C, by eating citrus fruits for vitamin C and nuts, bananas and berries for other nutrients including the B vitamins. If you add fresh salad as discussed, they will also provide you with vitamins and other nutrients. The salmon dinner, along with vegetables, salad, and 100% whole wheat dinner rolls should take about 25 to 30 minutes to prepare.

You can cook the mixed vegetables using your favorite recipe or according to the following recipe.

Ingredients for mixed vegetables;

- 4 teaspoonfuls of seasoned salt
- 3 cups of water
- 2 cups of broccoli
- 2 cups of mixed vegetables (Green beans, red and yellow sweet pepper, carrots, cauliflower and onions)
- 1 teaspoonful of garlic powder
- 1 teaspoonful of basil leaves
- ¾ teaspoonful of nutmeg
- ¾ teaspoonful of curry

- ¾ teaspoonful of black pepper
- 3 teaspoonfuls of fresh squeezed lemon

Place the water in a deep pot and add each of the seasonings except for the fresh squeezed lemon. Bring the water to a rapid boil. This would take about 10 to 15 minutes. In the meantime, wash the mixed vegetables and broccoli. Set them aside. When the seasoned water comes to a rapid boil, pour them into the pot. Mix well so that they are soaked in the fluid and turn off heat. Let stand in residual heat for two to three minutes, and then remove pot from heat. Add the fresh lemon juice directly to the fluid without allowing it to touch the vegetables. Mix well. Then remove the vegetables and serve immediately. The green beans and broccoli will look steamed and retain their green color. Do not overcook them. This will serve five to eight people.

Determine if you like them with or without fresh lemon juice. You can set aside one-half of the vegetables before adding lemon. Then taste the ones with lemon and ones without, to determine your preference.

Slice some delicious apples. Serve the salmon fillets along with the sliced apples, vegetables; as well as the salad. This should serve about six people. Serve with the 100% whole wheat dinner rolls (warm). Eat limited amount of the dinner rolls.

Procrastination

Some people want to live a healthy life. They know what they need to do to live a healthy life but they keep postponing taking the first step towards healthy living. They are uncomfortable with change. They have reasons why they cannot make changes each week. So these people keep waiting for a new year to make resolutions to live healthy and at the same time they keep breaking the resolution that they made in the past year. When people continue to procrastinate and fail to take steps towards healthy living, they are left to cheer and admire those who live a healthy lifestyle; and who look healthy. They say that their goal is to live a healthy lifestyle and look healthy and yet they do not implement the crucial steps necessary to make these a reality.

Suggestions for Procrastination

When procrastination stands in your way of a healthy lifestyle, remember Daniel whom I discussed earlier. Daniel started the right way and achieved desirable results. Successful healthy living does not start physically. It does not start with the things that you do or things that you did not do. It starts mentally. If you think the right thoughts, the right actions will follow naturally. Stop worrying about what you have not done or how difficult the things you need to do are. Remind yourself instead of the benefits you are trying to obtain through healthy living. Consider the long term benefits in appearance and health of implementing a healthy lifestyle. Make a determination to become healthier and then adhere to healthy choices. When you have made a determination, strengthen your determination with a commitment to do what you need to do to accomplish your goal. Get started right away with healthy living.

Lack of Accountability

Some people want to continue with their usual lifestyles. They believe that they are doing what they can to maintain a reasonable weight and be healthy. They do not want to be bordered by anyone about their weight and health. In this situation, one question becomes important. Can you remain healthy with your current weight situation and lifestyle in five years time? If the answer to this question is no then something different needs to be done.

Others believe that they are unable to change their lifestyle and that they are meant to live with unhealthy weight. They believe that nothing can be done about it. On the contrary, with the right modifications in lifestyle, a healthier weight is attainable. Some people just need more drastic measures than others and also more lifestyle modifications than others to achieve a healthy lifestyle along with a healthy weight.

Suggestions for Lack of Accountability

It is very helpful to commit to changes that will result in a healthy lifestyle and weight. It is equally important to have an accountability partner who cares about your healthy living goal and who will cheer you on to accomplish your goal. Incorporate healthy choices into your lifestyle and make those changes part of your daily life for a healthier you.

Desires

Some people have a reason why they eat every food or snack that they like and are accustomed to. They believe that they need them. You often hear a person in this situation say about a healthy food choice, "I can't eat this because I do not like it." They will also say, "This does not taste as good, it is too healthy." You will notice that a person who considers food in this way is most likely having problems with maintaining a healthy weight. They usually preserve in their diet foods with a lot of saturated fat that taste very good and foods that rapidly boost blood glucose level. They also continue to drink soft drinks or sodas daily. These foods and beverages sabotage good weight and good health in people who maintain them in their diet for frequent consumption.

When it comes to the choices of food and beverages that you surround yourself with, always think of the effect of eating such foods over time. Health and wellbeing are long term issues. You want to think of what would happen as years go by if you continue what you are doing.

Some people believe that they will eat what they want and work it out. Eventually, these people realize that they are unable to keep up with working out what they eat. They succumb to being overweight. They keep saying that they will do something about their weight and yet nothing changes. Over time weight becomes for them a source of frustration or even a cause for a depressed state.

Suggestions for Desires

If you find out that something that you like is capable of hurting you, there is a good chance that you will try to stay away from that thing. When it comes to your health, by the time you find out that something you like is very bad for you, it might be too late to avoid the ill health that it causes; and the consequences of the ill health. To be healthy, you need to be proactive about avoiding unhealthy indulgencies.amd put health above desire. Do not eat yourself to overweight and then struggle with weight loss. Search out healthy things that taste good. Drink water and limited 100 % juice daily. Making adjustments to accommodate healthy foods and beverages daily is crucial. They make good weight and good health easy to achieve. They also remove the frustration that can set in if one struggles with weight. It decreases your sources of daily stress. Prevention of damage is much better and easier than frantic efforts to control damage and recover from it.

Meal Course Orders (A Multi-Course Meal)

Many people who can achieve a healthy weight and live healthy lives are trapped in another hidden weight obstacle. This hidden obstacle is the non beneficial meal course orders. Healthy living and healthy weight are affected tremendously not just by what you eat but the way you eat. Some people know what they ought to eat. They even buy what they need to eat to be healthy but they eat the right food in the wrong order. A multi-course meal can consist of an appetizer, a side dish, a main dish, and a dessert. Unfortunately, without even noticing, some people eat foods with high glycemic index as appetizers and side dish. They also end up eating them as main dish and dessert. When they are full, they eat a minimal token amount of fruits and vegetables which make up less than 10% of their total meal. This type of eating, unfortunately, will only lead to weight increase rather than weight decrease. It will also lead to ill health rather than good health.

Suggestions for Meal Course Orders

Fruits and vegetables need to make up at least 55 % of the foods that you eat daily. This will tremendously benefit your health and weight. Eat them before your main dishes. This will allow you to obtain a lot of fiber which will help you feel fuller and enable you to eat less of the foods that would make you gain weight. Instead of having a spike in your blood sugar levels after you eat, you will have lower blood sugar levels which will decrease your risk of obesity and your risk of type II diabetes. It will also decrease your blood pressure. It will be extremely difficult to maintain good health and weight if fruits and vegetables are not significant sources of your daily calories. Weight loss as well as long term maintenance of a good weight will be much easier this way.

Avoid the mindset that you can enjoy your favorite foods everyday and work it out later. It is the easiest path to obesity. Those work-out routines you intend to do are necessary even when you are eating the right foods. They will not magically reverse the effects of eating less healthy foods over time. When someone is gaining weight daily, lifestyle modification becomes urgent.

Large Meal Portion Traditions

Some people come from families where delicious large portions of high glycemic foods are made and eaten every day. Usually in this situation, a lot of family members become overweight or obese. Over time, people in this situation believe that they are meant to be big and overweight. After all, everyone in the family is overweight. An example of this is where people are accustomed to having each family member eat a large plate full of spaghetti along with several white dinner rolls for dinner. Some even add a desert which has a high glycemic index. Anybody can become overweight with this type of dinners.

Some people are predisposed to obesity through their gene. Gene alone, however, does not guarantee manifestation of obesity. As a matter of fact, gene can serve as forewarning to motivate people to proactively avoid obesity.

Suggestions for Large Meal Portion Traditions

Reducing the portion size of your food is a very good idea. Spaghetti dinner is an example of food where people eat giant portions. One serving of spaghetti or a closed fist size of spaghetti is more than enough for one meal. This will occupy about one-fourth of a dinner plate. Fill the rest of the dinner plate with vegetables such as zucchini slices, broccoli, carrots or other vegetables of your choice. You can also have mushrooms and one serving of a clean fish. That will make almost three-fourth of dinner plate full of vegetables with fish. You can also eat nuts for protein. Simple modifications such as these will have huge impact in the health and weight of any family.

Take healthy living seriously in all aspects of life. Get some help if you need it. Avoid pitfalls that will sabotage your efforts.

The Love of Sugars and Candies

Some people love to eat generous amounts of sugar at every opportunity. This is not helpful towards good health. It is extremely difficult to eat a lot of sugar everyday and maintain good health and good weight at the same time. This is true whether the source of the sugar that is consumed is natural or not. Even when the right things towards good health and weight are done, unhealthy weight can persist due to these.

The worst comfort foods to eat are candies. Some people consider candies their "best friend" in hard times while in reality candies are their worst friend at all times. Some people have made candies part of their daily relaxation and have eaten themselves into obesity. When there is excess weight, some of the other diseases are enhanced. Some people gain up to seven pounds a week on candies alone. The candies sabotage their weight loss efforts and they wonder why they are not dropping the pounds in spite of efforts.

Consumption of generous amounts of candies can also be bad for your dental health. It boosts the activities of oral bacteria and it can increase the risk of developing cavities and other dental problems.

Suggestions for the Love of Sugars and Candies

Food labels indicate where there is generous amount of sugars and calories; a problem that can be avoided. If you love sugars and candies, there will be a need for you to re-evaluate their role in your health and weight. They can be a hindrance to healthy living efforts. There are a lot of delicious fresh, natural, and healthy alternatives to them. Use pure cane sugar to sweeten your food and use very limited amount. You can even omit sugar altogether and sweeten your foods using fresh crushed delicious fruits of your choice. You can also use fresh raw honey to sweeten foods. Making these changes in what you eat will yield dramatic results in your health and weight.

Reduce candy consumption to only once in a while. Consider eating candies only once in a month in very reduced portion. Be sure to floss and brush your teeth thoroughly before going to bed at night if you eat candy. This is necessary even when you eat limited amount of candy.

Financial Limitations: Limited Money for Healthy Food Purchase

Unfortunately, the inability to afford healthy foods can stand in the way of healthy eating. Fruits, vegetables, whole grains and healthy proteins which are recommended as healthy foods tend to be expensive for some people. Unhealthy processed foods and refined grains, on the other hand, are cheap and more affordable. Some families may find healthy foods difficult to afford.

Suggestions Concerning Financial Limitations

Affording recommended foods may need some planning in families where there are financial limitations. I have seen interesting results while looking at advertised food items from different stores, for over 10 years. Exactly the same item vary tremendously in prices in different stores or markets. If affordability is a concern for you, shop around and find places where the healthy items are cheaper. Compare prices from fruit and vegetable stands, tropical markets, large retail stores and whole sale stores which are open to the public. Shop when the grocery stores have a sale on the items that you need. Buy and stock-up on as many items as you are able to afford. Take advantage of the buy one get one free options. Also print out on-line coupons or use in-store coupons for your purchases. Shop also, at the end of holidays, to take advantage of holiday season sale for healthy foods. These foods include meats such as turkey after Thanksgiving and nuts after Christmas.

Fortunately, there are now dollar markets or shops where everything is a dollar. Some of these places have healthy food items for one dollar. These healthy food items include 100 % whole wheat bread, nuts such as almonds, and seeds. Window shop in these stores and see the natural whole foods that they have for sale. Avoid the junk foods that are sold in these places. Focus on the healthy food items only. Compare the size and price of the items to those in other stores.

Consider growing your own fruits and vegetables in your backyard. If you are unable to grow them in your backyard, try potted vegetables and fruits the same way you can grow potted flowers. Good quality large tomatoes, broccolis, cauliflower, green beans, onions, and berries can be grown in large flower pots at home. Some of these are grown and harvested in less than three months. Retail stores that sell potted plants as well as home and garden stores can give some good advice on how to grow these foods. They can be grown from seeds or as very young plants. This will help to make healthy fruits and vegetables more affordable.

Action Summary # 10: Part A

Be a part of positive influence instead of yielding to negative influence from your friends and co-workers. Suggest healthy foods with friends and associates for group dinners. Suggest weight loss competition. Avoid indulging in alcohol consumption and smoking with friends. Suggest healthier activities such as a ball game. As much as possible choose friends who will support healthy habits.

Strive to adhere to healthy choices that will help you to maintain good health. Avoid poor health choices even if it is promoted in your environment. Avoid watching hours of television and eating unhealthy foods and snacks with television.

Practice good oral hygiene and get good dental attention. Consistent bad breath could be an indication of poor dental health. Floss your teeth daily. Cleaning the tongue thoroughly is also very helpful. Adhere to good oral hygiene Practice good sleeping hygiene to facilitate your sleep at night. Lack of sufficient sleep can result in poor health.

Finish your exercise four to five hours before bedtime. Do a relaxing activity to alleviate stress before going to bed. Avoid alcohol close to bedtime because even though you can fall asleep with alcohol intake, you will not be rested. Avoid stimulants such as caffeine around bedtime. When in a different time zone, sleep as close to your regular time zone as you can. Decrease late night outings to allow for better rest at night. Try to resolve bothersome issues or talk to someone you trust to help alleviate worry and discouragement and be able to sleep at night.

Avoid eating quick unhealthy foods due to a busy schedule. Start making quick healthy dinners which include salmon. We saw some examples of this in this chapter. Avoid using aluminum foil in baking food or covering hot food. Commit to healthy living and involve an accountability partner to support you. Not everything we desire is good for us. Do not be led by your desires. Change what you do and what you eat to what is good for your health and weight.

Avoid foods with high glycemic index. Allow vegetables and some fruits to make up at least 55 % of your food. Reduce the portion size of your foods and make up the missing portion with vegetables and fruits. Avoid candies and sugars. Use fresh fruits or honey sometimes to sweeten foods. If you have limited resources shop in discount stores and grow your vegetables.

Part B

Stress and Disease States

Stress

Stress is a normal response of the body to demands in our lives. It increases when we have difficulty with situations around us and decreases when we have our situations under control. When stress is constant and unmanaged it becomes a threat to good health.

There are various situations that cause stress for people every day. Traffic causes stress. Examinations cause stress for students. Some people have financial stress. Taking care of the family can be a source of stress. Holiday shopping stress can be a significant problem for some people. Work is a source of stress for many people as well.

The body responds to stress by making certain changes. Stress causes the body to release certain hormones. Hormones released in the body during stress include adrenaline and cortisol. Adrenaline energizes you. Adrenaline also increases your heart rate. It helps to prepare you for response to your situation. Cortisol increases blood glucose levels. Cortisol also enhances the efficiency of the use of glucose by the brain. The body is also prepared for response in other ways. All these changes brought about in the body affect you in such a way as to enable you to response to your situation. Cortisol is the major stress hormone. When you are no longer stressed, the levels of adrenaline and cortisol fall. Your heart rate returns to normal and your blood glucose level decreases. If you are constantly under stress, the continual release of stress hormones can put you at risk for a number of diseases.

Stress Related Disease States

Constant stress increases your risk for the following diseases states or problems;

- Hypertension (High blood Pressure)

- Heart disease
- Insomnia
- Overweight and obesity
- Digestive problems
- Skin problems and break-outs
- Depression
- Problems with memory
- Alopecia or hair loss

Stress and Hair

What does Stress Have to do with Hair?

Stress plays havoc with the hair. This effect on the hair is usually not apparent to the person under stress. Over time the hair gets eroded. I have seen some people go from having bountiful hair to barely having any hair at all due to severe sustained stress.

Alopecia, which is hair loss, can result as a direct consequence of stress. When someone has severe stress the hair can stop growing and thriving and stay dormant. If the stress is sustained, portions of the hair will fall out during combing, washing, or while having a hair relaxer treatment.

Suggestions for Stress

Stress can be managed. Recognize the sources of your stress and try to minimize your stress. The best way to eliminate traffic stress is to plan to get to your destination one hour in advance. When you arrive at your destination, do something relaxing if the traffic allows you to arrive at your destination one hour prior to your scheduled function. Listen to music, observe nature or just sit back and relax prior to starting your work or event. This will allow you to start your work or event without undue stress. If on the other hand you experience traffic delay, the one hour extra time that you have allowed will be enough to allow most traffic delays to clear. This will allow you to still get to your function on time without unnecessary stress. The greatest advantage of this type of planning is the relative peace of mind that you will have while in traffic. You will not have to worry about your blood pressure increasing due to traffic stress. You will be calm knowing that the chance of arriving at your destination on time is very high.

The best way to reduce examination stress is to make sure that you complete each day's studying and homework assignment the same day your lecture is given. Make sure you understand your topics and get help promptly when needed to enable you to complete your homework assignments correctly. Never postpone any studying or home work till the next day. When in examination hall, having prepared well, remind yourself that you have worked hard and that the examination material ought not to be a strange concept to you. Take a couple of deep breaths and relax before you start taking your examination.

When there are financial difficulties, reducing expenses can help to stretch one's resources to meet financial obligations. In some cases this may be sufficient to address the problem. If financial difficulties persist, in spite of reduced expenses, consider self improvement for better earning. Also consider relocating to a place with better jobs. Sometimes relocation may be necessary to obtain a desired outcome for you and your family.

Some of the stresses that come with taking care of the family can be reduced. Young moms taking care of young children at home or home schooling their children can get together with other moms in similar situations and participate in group activities to reduce stress. People taking care of adult family members can join a support group of people who have similar circumstances and who encourage each other and reduce stress through mutual support.

To reduce holiday shopping stress, spread out your holiday shopping times throughout the year. You can even take advantage of the Christmas clearance once Christmas is over. You can start shopping for the next Christmas gifts with these sales. Continue shopping, periodically, till Christmas. This will give you plenty of time to shop stress free, as well as allow you to save a lot of money due to clearance sales. Be sure to shop with a list of all the people you usually give Christmas gifts to. Put a check mark beside the names of people on your list after you purchase gifts for them. In addition to saving you money and reducing your stress, this will also free up time for you around Christmas and further reduce stress.

Have a plan to help reduce the stress from your work. The plan could be as simple as having a long warm relaxing shower after work every day. If you have access to a Jacuzzi, you can have a Jacuzzi bath after work also. Be sure to use for the shower or Jacuzzi, moisturizing and pleasantly smelling shower gel or bath crystal. Follow this with a good moisturizing cream or lotion.

Taking a walk around the neighborhood can also be helpful. Any relaxing activity which can help to reduce your stress is helpful after work whether you work outside the home or not.

Laughter for Stress Relief

Get some daily laughter into your life. Laughing even when you are not in a very good situation can tremendously reduce your stress. You can read a funny book. Your local library will have a lot of funny books. You can find clean jokes or shows that can make you laugh. Even some TV preachers can make you laugh a lot. Just 15 to 30 minutes of TV is more than enough for you to get your laugh. This is not an invitation to become a couch potato or a TV addict because spending hours in front of the TV is bad for your health.

Relaxation and Stress Reduction through Vivid Imagination or Visualization

You can decrease your stress by using vivid imaginations. I have seen vivid imaginations work successfully to reduce stress. You can imagine that you are back on a nature reserve, a beautiful park, a cruise, or any place that you thoroughly enjoyed. Create in your head a detailed and vivid image of this place. Think of its beauty and the delight it gave. Remember the delightful (and hopefully) healthy things you ate in this place and how enjoyable it was. Think of the sights and sounds you enjoyed in this place. Imagine a stretch of nature, the smell of wild flowers, and the sound of birds. Remember the squirrels, bunnies, and chipmunks that ran around and chased each other. Imagine the sight of a stretch of beach, the interesting shells on the beach, and the feel of sand on your feet. Imagine the sound of splashing waves. Just think of any experience that delighted your many senses and these will encourage you, make you smile, and alleviate stress.

Reducing stress is a vital part of staying healthy. When your daily stress is reduced, your chances of developing stress related diseases will decrease as well.

Negative Impact and Negative Thinking

Some degree of negative experiences seems to be common for many people. Unfortunately, some people have many negative experiences and these people have been impacted negatively in significant ways in their lives. Having a lot of negative experiences and reflecting on them frequently can adversely affect your good health. Some people have negative experiences from their jobs, schools, neighborhood, vacations, and even proms.

Negative experiences can make people to begin to think negatively. It can even become tempting for some people to always expect the worst because of past negative experiences. Expecting the worst may seem like a way to protect oneself from disappointment. However over time, negative thinking diminishes energy, increases stress, increases anxiety, and diminishes wellbeing. Some people may have been treated inappropriately and told that they cannot succeed in their endeavor. This may have to do with school, the use of their talent, or their desired career.

Suggestions for Negative Impact and Negative Thinking

Negative things which you cannot control can happen. The best thing that you can do for yourself is to ensure that you are not controlled by your negative experiences. They have served as a stepping-stone for some people. Negative circumstances and experiences have forced some people out of their comfort zone to a much better place in life. Some people have lost their stressful jobs, for instance, and then ended up in dream jobs. Others have lost their jobs and ended up starting and heading successful enterprises.

A lot of negative impacts end up having insignificant effect on your life in the long run. I once encountered some rather negative people, when I was younger, in the university during my first degree. I had to do some of the school work with them. I was concerned about that situation. I talked to my older sister, Dr.

Mercy Offor, about it. She told me to interact in the best way that I could with them but not to worry about them. She then said something that was very helpful and very important. She told me to remember that in a few years after I leave the school, whatever those people did or did not do will be in the past and virtually insignificant in my future life. She was right and it was exactly true. If I had continued to focus on and worry about it, I may have diminished my wellbeing over something that will end up having negligible significance in my life. When it comes to negative impact, do not focus on the here and now aspect of the situation. Your life has a bigger picture than any particular negative situation or impact.

Some people have been impacted negatively and told that they cannot succeed in their life's endeavors. These people have gone ahead and excelled in their endeavors and proved their critics wrong. I had to ignore critics to reach milestones in my life. You need to believe in God and yourself and not in your critics. Do not allow negative impact to occupy any significant position in your thought and life. Talk to people that care about you concerning negative issues that bother you. Talk to people who have their lives under control. Then make new plans and move on.

Never lose hold of positive thinking. Positive thinking will enhance your life, health, and relationships. Reflect on positive experiences as often as you can. Continue to be optimistic in your life. Optimism enhances wellbeing. Moses sent out twelve spies to spy out a new territory. Ten out of twelve spies were terrified of problems dealing with the giants in that area and they talked negatively about their chances of success and believed that they cannot succeed. They defeated themselves in their minds by so doing. Having already defeated themselves in their minds they, "brought up an evil report." They said negative things like, "We be not able to go up against the people; for they are stronger than we," and, "we saw the giants." They also said, "And we were in our own sight as grasshoppers, and so we were in their sight." See Numbers 13: 31-33 (KJV).

Negative thinking can deplete the energy needed for progress. Joshua and Caleb two of the twelve spies kept hope and optimism alive. Joshua and Caleb saw major obstacles ahead of them in the form of giants who were much bigger than them physically. They acknowledged the giants but refused to be afraid of them. Caleb said, "Let us go up at once, and possess it; for we are well able to overcome it," Numbers 13: 30 (KJV)). This is in spite of the fact that 10 of their peers only looked at the problems and not the possibility of solutions. Their peers listed terrifying obstacles including the strengths of their opponents.

Joshua and Caleb were optimistic and talked positively about their situation. They needed to take over the land of those giants. They believed that they could do it not by themselves but through God's help. Joshua and Caleb's positive thinking and confession brought success, because they trusted God when the situation was beyond them. Asking for God's help is the best thing that you can do when situations are beyond you and out of your control. You have nothing to lose. Some people say that there is no soldier who does not believe in God at the moment when death seems inevitable in wars. God has unusual ways of solving impossible problems. Joshua and Caleb's dependence of God caused them to succeed in the end in spite of enormous legitimate obstacles.

Stay in touch with people who can encourage you. Positive people impart energy and also empower you. Encouragement is a very helpful aspect of a healthy mind. My brother, Dan, a published author who heads a department, epitomizes encouragement. He is our only brother out of eight children. He offers such heartwarming encouragement to us. Sometimes it is simply rejuvenating. So definitely associate with an encourager to help nullify the negative impacts that you experience.

Unforgiveness

Sometimes caterpillars invade small plants as well as trees and attempt to eat up their leaves. Incidentally some people function like 'human caterpillars' to offend and wear other people out. People can cause offence in all kinds of ways. Sometimes some people, for some reason, actually invest time and efforts into things that they know could cause other people pain. These offences can occur anywhere including school and work. You usually will remember what people have done to offend you. You can even remember the details that they may have forgotten.

It is natural to want to hold accountable those who have offended you. Bearing grudges is part of the attempt to hold people accountable for what they have done to you. Some people actually believe that not holding unto offences committed against them is condoning the offences. They remember, rehash, and experience over and over the offences and the pain. Each time the body responds to the intense negative emotion resulting in the increase in heart rate and blood pressure. Bearing grudges can therefore affect the cardiovascular system. Bearing grudges can increase stress and cause the muscles to become tensed especially those in the neck and shoulder. This can result in pain in the neck and shoulders. The stress can also result in headache. Some people attempt to treat these with over-the-counter medications while holding onto the source of pain. This can results in a viscous cycle.

The worst thing about grudge is that people could have a grudge and insist sincerely that they do not have it. That is until they see their offender or have to talk about their offender. They will call them names in anger or confront them when they have the opportunity concerning the past offence. One way to test whether you are free from grudge is to note how you feel about your offender, the offence; and how you talk about them. You are free from grudges if you could talk about the offenders without any rising anger

243

Suggestions for Unforgiveness

The first thing that is important to understand about forgiveness is that forgiving people does not mean that you are excusing, condoning, or even forgetting what they have done. It simply means that you are fully aware of what they have done but you are choosing to become free from the burdens which accompany grudge, anger, and resentment. You will not realize the weight that will be lifted off of you until you fully forgive and completely let go of the offence. Some people do not deserve to be forgiven but you need to forgive them anyway.

Patience and forgiveness go together. If you become patient with people it will be easier to forgive them. Human nature and human interactions leave a lot of room for offence. One of the best things you can do for your health is to have a plan to forgive those who have offended you and those who will offend you. Do not surround yourself with people who are negative and offensive in their ways. If you encounter them, however, extend forgiveness to them. Some people live negative and miserable lives and that is all they know. They cannot give what they do not have to other people.

If you forgive people who have offended you, they will only be able to hurt you in a minimal way. If you are unable to forgive them, on the other hand, they will end up hurting you more in the long run as unforgiveness can adversely affect your health. You cannot be emotionally healthy if you are unable to forgive people who have offended you. Poor emotional health over time diminishes overall health.

Forgiveness is more powerful and more beneficial than revenge. Some people are engaged in a battle of revenge. They revenge on their enemies and their enemies revenge on them. Each party is occupied with plans for revenge and in the whole pursuit; peace is completely lost by both parties. All the people that are involved with this, end up with diminished health in the process. I have discussed forgiveness with primary care physicians. For certain situations the health of patients improves when they forgive their offenders. When you forgive people you are not letting the offenders run wild. Not forgiving those who have offended you is like wrestling someone to the floor and holding that person so that he or she will not get back up. All the while you are holding the person to the floor you are not free either. You may have the satisfaction of holding them down to the floor but you lose your freedom in the process.

The offenders may seem free but they are really not free. It is sometimes like dictators who hurt people repeatedly and seem invincible. Sooner or later their dictatorship come to an end and some of them suffer what they made other people suffer through the years. Let offences go and pursue positive living and better health.

Unforgiveness is a burden too heavy for anyone to carry and also a health hazard. There is a liberating freedom along with healing that comes with forgiveness and letting go of offences. It is hard to believe but easy and wonderful to experience.

Benefits of Forgiveness

- Improved emotional health
- Reduced stress
- Better cardiovascular health
- Decreased muscle tension and pain
- Improved overall health

Lack of Self Acceptance

Some people have been made to feel so bad about who they are that they are unable to accept themselves. Other people actually give them the impression that as long as they remain the way they are made they will not be accepted. These people are not telling them to be better or improve. They actually want them to become somebody else to be accepted; which is impossible. In other words they are made to feel that because they are not somebody else something is wrong with them. Some people actually tell other people that they are not success material either as far as school is concerned or as far as a career is concerned.

Suggestions for Lack of Self Acceptance

You are unique and there is no one else in the world like you. You have abilities that are unique to you and you can make a contribution to life that no one else can make. Be the best that you can be, stay around positive people, and say no to the influences and manipulations of negative people.

Remember that you are not who negative people want you to think that you are. Some people are trapped in a negative mindset and the problem is with them, not with you. Separate yourself from negative people. Do not worry about those who refuse to love you. They may not love themselves either. This is important because you need to have a healthy mind along with a healthy body for optimal health.

Some community organizations provide support groups that encourage people. They try to connect people with those that care about them. The support and encouragement help diffuse stress. Get connected with a positive group of people as soon as you can.

Remember that your destiny is not determined by what people say or how people perceive you. Some people were told that they are not the type that can succeed and they ended up succeeding and having national or international impact.

If it is possible, travel to an international destination. See how other people live. Perform some research on cultures other than yours. Ask questions about other cultures to enable you to choose a place that will be rewarding. International travel helps to broaden someone's perspective on life and most often in a positive way. Some people have found so much happiness in their international trips that they have made room eventually to have a vacation home in the places that they visited.

Protect yourself from falsehood and narrow minded opinions that can adversely affect how you feel about yourself. Over time these crucial steps towards healthier mind will be very rewarding with regards to your overall health. Healthy minds are important for optimal health.

Lack of Confidence

Certain cultures have embedded in them patterns of interaction that eventually erode people's confidence. Young children in such places are made to feel that they are not important because they are not friends with certain people around them. Others are made to feel unimportant because they do not have certain things that people around them have. These children as they become older are insulted and bullied even for things that they cannot control. By adulthood, their confidence gets diminished and some of them even become depressed. Unfortunately, some even commit suicide.

In cultures with better quality of life, young people are made to understand that in life, it is not where you started that is important or how you started but how you finished. This type of believe motivates people to strive to better themselves and achieve big things in life even if they started with a lot of disadvantages and little hope. This expectation for a better life than where they started, boost the confidence of young people and motivates them to ignore their current disadvantages and work hard for a better situation than they started with. In such cultures examples abound of people who have accomplished great things from very humble and disadvantaged beginnings. These examples further serve as motivation for young people with humble beginnings or disadvantages. In these types of cultures quality of life is generally high and people are happy and hopeful even when they are poor and have very little of what they need in life. Also people who have succeeded help people who are very needy.

Suggestions for Lack of Confidence

One of life's treasures is the ability to cling unto hope. Young people all over the world ought to know that not having certain people as friends and not having certain things at some stage in their lives are not indications of the type of people they will become. Working hard and staying focused can help people move forward in life. You cannot control how other people act but you can determine to stay focused and put in your best in everything that you are doing. With focus and hard work you could end up in a much better place in life than could ever be predicted from where you started. Having hope make people less vulnerable to lack of confidence, self pity and depression. Feeling that they could work toward changing their lives empower people to strive to achieve big things in life. Some people through hard work and focus end up in much better positions in life than their peers who had all the desirable things and friends earlier in life.

Isolation

Certain circumstances can cause some people to become isolated. When people are isolated, they are unable to get the encouragement that they need. They are unable to connect with the people who are going through the same thing as they are. They are unable to take advantage of support. Isolation is not a healthy situation. It is detrimental to the mind and to mental health.

Suggestions for Isolation

Try as much as you can to stay connected to other people. Seek out people that share your believe and interest and stay connected with those people. Avoid stressful social environment. Negative social environment is as unhealthy as isolation and can adversely affect your health. Surround yourself with a positive environment. You could even volunteer for a noble cause and stay in touch with people who are making a difference in other people's lives.

Whenever you are able go to your local library and read a few good books and learn something new. The local library, though full of people, can be a peaceful place to spend time sometimes. As a result of great technological progress there are numerous ways to stay connected with people on-line these days. There are even video call options that are available for communication on-line; face-to-face. Take advantage of these options and connect with the people of your choice. Technology has turned the world into a global community. You can now have friends from all over the world and can see and talk to them through on-line video calls.

Depressed State (Discouragement)

Some people already know the right activities to participate in and the right food to eat to be healthy. However, they often deviate from the healthy food and activities that they are used to; when they are discouraged or when they are in a depressing situation. Some people eat generous amount of regular crust pizzas, potato chips, or ice cream when they are in a depressing situation. Eating generous amount of these can result in rapid weight gain. It can even increase the risk of ill health in many ways.

Unfortunately, the worst thing a person can do to a depressed state is to eat unhealthy foods. This is the case because unhealthy foods, when they increase weight, might result in ill health as well as health related expenses. All of these might put the person in a worsened state of depression. It, therefore, becomes a cycle of depressed state where the action due to a depressed state results ultimately in another depressed state. An example of this is a situation where repeated consumption of unhealthy foods due to a depressed state result in sustained hyperglycemia (high blood glucose) and a possible trip to the emergency room. The emergency room sometimes can be busy and the wait to be seen can be long and frustrating in spite of good efforts from the healthcare workers. The scare and the frustration from this experience and the lost time can lead to another depressed state. If eating unhealthy is chosen as a way out of a depressed state, the danger of ill health might be repeated or obesity can occur. It is like "jumping from a hot frying pan into an open fire." Trust me; you do not want to go from bad to worse.

Suggestions Concerning Depressed State

I have been around people who have gone through tough and discouraging situations and found successful ways of recovering from their adverse circumstances. If you are in a depressed state due to your circumstances, consider the following measures instead of unhealthy eating:

- Healthy snacking
- Spending time in a scenic park, garden or nature reserve
- Long walk along the beach
- Write a very positive journal
- Working on a long standing project
- Window shopping in an outdoor mall
- Change of environment

Healthy Snacking in a Discouraged or Depressed State

If you must eat when you are discouraged, choose delicious deep colored grapes, some nuts such as almonds, or seeds. These can be delicious and there could be some comfort in the prolonged chewing that go with eating these healthy snacks. Some fruits such as cherries, blueberries, blackberries and vegetables such as carrots are very delicious. You can sample them and see which of these fruits and vegetables you find delicious. Some people snack on bran cereal with added fresh fruits. Eating any of these suggested foods may not feel right initially but when you persist and remember that they will improve your health and appearance it will be worthwhile. Over time, it will feel good and rewarding to eat something that will not adversely affect your health during times of discouragement. They will increase your fiber intake. Your health will improve in the process rather than deteriorate and you could lose rather than gain weight. All these will result in your being encouraged at the end rather than the other way around.

Spend limited time staying around food and eating. Do not feel trapped with food. Varying your activity when discouraged is beneficial. Interrupt the eating session by opting to get away for some time.

Spending Time in a Scenic Park, Garden or Nature Reserve

Being indoors during a time of discouragement can exacerbate your discouraged state of mind. The beauty of nature can sometimes be very uplifting and can boost your mood. You can spend time in or walk around a scenic park and enjoy its beauty. If you have access to a garden spend some time there or take a walk around it. Watch the squirrels run around or the birds fly around. You can also walk around a nature reserve. You will be surrounded by nature and can take advantage of the calming feeling that nature gives. These exposures to nature can take your mind away from your unpleasant situation. It might even allow you to think clearly and come up with a solution for some of your situations.

Long Walk Along the Beach

If you can get to the beach, spend some time there. Opt to do something relaxing while you are there. You can take a long walk there and enjoy nature all around the beach. You can even jog along the beach for some time.

Write a Very Positive Journal

Write about the compliments you have received, your accomplishments, your wise and profitable decisions and the contributions that you have made. Also write about the stories of people who have made it through adversity.

Sometimes when you are discouraged, you can forget how you have made a difference in one area or the other. You can forget how you made it through a hard situation. You can even forget about a story that you have heard about someone who went through what you are going through and found a way out; or got some help along the way that got them out of the situation. You forget that with a little help you can get back on track. Recalling and journaling about these things can help you keep your focus despite your situation. It can also renew your confidence and help steer your mind towards a solution rather than succumb to a state of helplessness.

Working on a Long-Standing Project

You may be asking, "How can someone work to relieve discouragement?" Sometimes with our busy lifestyles we have something that we want to do but are unable to find time to do it. This could range from rearranging our closets to planting a garden. Who wants to settle down and work on a project discouraged or depressed? Working on something that you have postponed for a long time is the last thing you want to think about when you are discouraged or depressed. Completing a long-standing task, however, can boost your mood. You will have a great sense of accomplishment when you finally get the pending project taken care of.

Window-Shopping in an Outdoor Mall

"You must be joking," you might say. "Why should I waste my time going window-shopping?" Going window-shopping in an outdoor mall can actually save you shopping time eventually and in the meantime it can be a good distraction from a discouraged state of mind. You can go into the department store to examine the items that you like or verify their prices. This is not supposed to be an encouragement to go on a shopping spree. The great thing about window-shopping is that you are not under pressure to buy anything. As a matter of fact, it is best if you do not buy anything during window-shopping. It allows you to see what is new and how much they cost. When you are ready to shop, you can target clothes and other items that you already saw and liked. This can even make your shopping less stressful because you have an idea of the best place for each of the items that you need when you need them.

If I am close to the mall, I usually stop and do some window-shopping. Once in a while I go out just to be able to do some window-shopping. I started this mainly because I always had too little time to shop and when I finally get to it or when I am forced to shop to give gifts I get overwhelmed going frantically from one department store to another. I even get stressed out especially if I am not finding suitable items to purchase. Window-shopping has simplified my shopping so much that my gift giving is virtually free from stress. Window-shopping in an outdoor mall also gives you a good walking opportunity because you walk everywhere and without elevators, especially if you park your car at one end of the mall.

Change of Environment

If discouragement persists and every effort fails to lift you out of it, try to change your environment. Change is sometimes worthwhile. In extreme cases relocation has helped some people out of being in a discouraged state frequently. Relocation has changed some people's lives in a positive way. They went from struggling daily emotionally to actually being happy. Obviously this takes research of the places of interest. It also takes a visit to anywhere you desire to make sure that it will meet your needs. The places that you have visited or lived in before will obviously need no research if chosen.

Fear

Some people are afraid of failure so they do not even bother to take steps towards healthy living. Some people have tried some weight loss diets in the past, lost weight, and then gained back all the lost weight. They believe that it is no use trying to live healthy and lose weight since they will end up gaining the weight back. Some people even believe that healthy living will work for other people but will not work for them. They cheer other people on towards healthy living while succumbing to fear of failure and excluding themselves from participating in healthy living. It is important to remember that adopting a weight loss or diet plan is different from adopting a healthy lifestyle. Adopting a healthy lifestyle involves changing the way you live and doing things differently every day. It is like changing direction and following a new direction that naturally leads to a particular destination; which includes good health and a good weight.

Some people are afraid of failure because no one around them is living a healthy lifestyle. They believe that everyone around them is doing the same thing and that if change to a healthy lifestyle was attainable the people around them will be living healthy lifestyles.

Suggestions for Fear

Healthy living is completely different from a diet plan. Healthy living is basically lifestyle modifications that include healthy choices and actions that result in a healthier life. It involves adding certain things to your life and removing certain things from your life permanently. When you do that, you become healthier, look better, and have more energy. Your living healthier will result in weight loss. Forget whatever you have done in the past that was not successful. Forget about other people who are not living a healthy lifestyle. Do not look for people who live healthy and look good. Make up your mind to become that person who will live healthy and look good. Determine to commit to and continue with healthy choices and win with desirable outcome. You can go from leading the cheer in healthy living to leading the way in healthy lifestyle. Determination and commitment will get you there and you can enjoy the numerous benefits of good health.

Action Summary # 10: Part B

Recognize the causes of stress in your life and minimize your stress. Stress related diseases include: obesity, insomnia, heart disease, hypertension, skin problems and memory problems. Leave home earlier than is necessary for your event or work to help minimize traffic stress. Participate in a relaxing activity after work to help reduce work stress. Get connected with people who are in similar situations as you to help reduce family stress or join support groups. Complete daily homework assignments on the day they are assigned if you are a student to help reduce stress.

Stay optimistic even if you have been impacted negatively. Negative thinking increases stress and anxiety and diminishes health. You cannot control the negative things that happen to you. You can, however, refuse to allow them to control you. Your critics do not have the final say. Do not evaluate your worth by what negative people say about you. Some people have excelled academically and in careers that they have been told that they could not succeed in. Stay positive. Connect with people who can encourage you and move forward.

Forgive your offenders and preserve your health. Forgiveness has many health benefits. Some people have been told that they are not desirable. Do not lose your confidence no matter how certain people perceive you. You are unique and can make unique contribution to society. Do not get isolated. Stay connected with positive people.

Avoid becoming a victim of comfort food when you get discouraged. Spend time in profitable and relaxing activities. Write a very positive journal or work on a long-standing project that can give you relief and a boost in your mood. These will distract you from your discouragement. If you must eat when discouraged, eat healthier snacks such as all natural nuts, seeds, and fruits. Do not let the fear of failure keep you from adopting a healthy lifestyle.

Chapter Eleven

Vitamins

Basic understanding of vitamins is useful towards healthy living. It will enrich your food choices. Vitamins are involved in various growth processes and they enable the body to function efficiently. The important roles that they play in our bodies enhance good health. It is very important to ensure that these nutrients are not depleted in the body.

When the levels of the vitamins needed by the body are low, the functions of the body can become compromised. Healthy eating improves dramatically the chance of obtaining the daily required vitamins. A few of them are available in fortified foods.

As you broaden the healthy foods that you eat, especially the deep colored natural fresh foods; you will obtain a wide range of these needed nutrients. This will minimize symptoms of deficiencies or even illness.

They help to protect the body against diseases and cancers. Vitamins are obtained usually from the diet. The body however, is able to make vitamin D. Vitamin D is made in the skin using ultraviolet light from sunlight. So vitamin D production requires exposure to the sun. I will discuss some vitamins briefly.

People sometimes develop a vitamin deficiency. Deficiency of vitamins can result in a number of medical conditions. If you have a vitamin deficiency, your doctor will help you determine the amount that you need to take to help resolve the deficiency. Vitamins are either fat soluble or water soluble.

Vitamins include the following:

- Vitamin A
- Vitamin B1
- Vitamin B2
- Vitamin B3
- Vitamin B5
- Vitamin B6
- Vitamin B7
- Vitamin B9
- Vitamin B12
- Vitamin C
- Vitamin D
- Vitamin E
- Vitamin K

Vitamin A (Retinol, Retinal and Carotenoids, Beta-Carotene)

Vitamin A is fat soluble. It is available from plants and animals. It is available from plants sources, as carotenoids. Carotenoids are provitamins. Vitamin A which is obtained from animal sources is retinoid. Retinoid is the preformed vitamins A. Carotenoids like beta-carotene have the most vitamin A activity. Vitamin A is absorbed in the form of retinol.

The deficiency of vitamin A results in the following:

- Vision problems and in extreme cases blindness
- Vulnerability to infections
- Skin problems

Vitamin A plays very important roles in vision. It also enhances bone growth. It helps to boost the immune system. It is very beneficial for good health. Beta-carotene has antioxidant properties against damage causing free radicals.

Healthy sources of vitamin A include:

- Broccoli
- Blackberries
- Cantaloupe
- Carrots
- Green leafy vegetables such as spinach and collard greens
- Mango
- Papaya
- Sweet potato
- Eggs
- Milk
- Whole grain cereals

Is There Any Harm with Vitamin A?

Provitamin A carotenoids such as beta-carotene are generally considered safe because they are not associated with specific adverse health effects (1). Their conversion to vitamin A decreases when body stores are full (1). A high intake of provitamin A carotenoids can turn the skin yellow, but this is not considered dangerous to health (1).

You do not have to worry about problems with vitamin A from food sources, unless you eat liver in excess. If you are taking vitamin A supplements, toxicity and problems can occur with too much vitamin A supplementation.

Excess vitamin A supplement intake can result in symptoms that include headache and dry skin. Prolonged intake of excess amount of this vitamin supplements can result in symptoms that include vision problems. Excess vitamin A supplement has adverse effect on bones also. This can increase the risk of bone fracture.

Daily Required Amount of Vitamin A

The daily required amount of vitamin A is as follows:

Males 14 years of age and older require about 3,000 IU or 900 mcg per day

Females 14 years of age and older requires about 2,300 IU or about 650 mcg per day

Pregnant females will need up to 2,500 IU or 750 mcg per day

Nursing mothers need about 4,100 IU or about 1,250 mcg

Vitamin B1 (Thiamine)

Vitamin B1 is water soluble. It is involved with the breakdown of foods such as carbohydrates into glucose. The glucose is then used for energy production. It enhances healthy skin and hair. Deficiency of vitamin B1 results in Beriberi and a brain disorder.

Healthy sources of vitamin B1 include:

- Nuts
- Seeds
- Oats
- Whole grain cereal
- Wheat
- Oranges
- Milk
- Beans
- Lentils

Daily Required Amount of Vitamin B1

The daily required amount of vitamin B1 is as follows:

Males 14 years of age and older require about 1.3 mg per day

Females 14 years of age and older requires about 1.0 mg per day

Pregnant females and nursing mothers will need about 1.5 mg per day

Vitamin B2 (Riboflavin)

Vitamin B2 is water soluble. It is involved with the breakdown of foods such as carbohydrates. The glucose which results from the breakdown of carbohydrate is used to produce energy. It enhances healthy skin and hair. Deficiency manifestations include skin problems and cracks at the corners of the mouth. Some people have used it to alleviate headache.

Healthy sources of vitamin B2 include:

- Almonds
- Bran cereal
- Broccoli
- Cauliflower
- Milk
- Mushroom
- Orange juice (Orange juice is not a major source of riboflavin)

Daily Required Amount of Vitamin B2

The daily required amount of vitamin B2 is as follows:

Males 14 years of age and older require about 1.6 mg per day
Females 14 years of age and older requires about 1.2 mg per day

Pregnant females and nursing mothers will need about to 1.6 mg per day

Vitamin B3 (Niacin, Niacinamide, Nicotinic Acid)

Vitamin B3 is water soluble. It is involved with the breakdown of foods such as carbohydrates for energy production. It enhances the maintenance of a healthy digestive system. It is useful for healthy skin and hair. Deficiency of vitamin B3 results in Pellagra. Pellagra is very well known because of its four classic symptoms all of which begin with the letter 'D'. I call them the pellagra "D's". Pellagra symptoms are; dermatitis, diarrhea, dementia and death.

Healthy sources include:

- Avocados
- Bran cereal
- Cereal grains
- Green vegetable
- Fish such as salmon
- Seeds such as pumpkin seeds
- Chicken (contains an amino acid, tryptophan which the liver converts into niacin)
- Eggs (contains the amino acid, tryptophan also)
- Milk (contains the amino acid, tryptophan as well)

Daily Required Amount of Vitamin B3

The daily required amount of vitamin B3 is as follows:

Males 14 years of age and older require about 16 mg per day
Females 14 years of age and older requires about 14 mg per day
Pregnant females and nursing mothers will need about 17 mg per day

Vitamin B5 (Pantothenic Acid)

Vitamin B5 is water soluble. It is involved with the breakdown of foods such as carbohydrates for energy production. It enhances healthy skin and hair. Deficiency of vitamin B5 result in a number of problems including: Fatigue, burning feet and paresthesia (tingling and numbness sensation). Vitamin B5 enhances wound healing and acne reduction. Pantothenic acid comes from the word pantothen, which means everywhere or from every side. This vitamin is available from numerous plants and animal sources.

Healthy sources include:

- Avocados
- Broccoli
- Cauliflower
- Legumes
- Tomato
- Fish such as salmon
- Poultry

- Eggs
- Whole grain

Some people use Pantothenic acid to help them with conditions that include: Acne, baldness, grey hair, osteoarthritis, rheumatoid arthritis, carpal tunnel syndrome and burning feet.

Daily Required Amount of Vitamin B5

The daily required amount of vitamin B5 is as follows:

Teens and adults require about 5 mg per day
Pregnant females and nursing mothers will need about 6 mg per day

Vitamin B6 (Pyridoxine, Pyridoxamine)

Vitamin B6 is water soluble. It has six forms. Two of these forms of vitamin B6 are the active coenzyme forms. It is involved with the breakdown of foods such as carbohydrates for the production of energy. It is useful for healthy skin and hair.

The deficiency of vitamin B6 results in a variety of problems including:

- Anemia
- Cracks at the corners of the mouth
- Lowered immune function

The two active coenzyme forms of vitamin B6 are pyridoxal 5'
phosphate (referred to as PLP) and pyridoxamine 5' phosphate
(referred to as PMP). These two coenzymes, PLP and PMP, are the
forms of vitamin B6 that are involved in numerous reactions in the
body. These numerous reactions have to do with protein
metabolism in the body. PLP is involved with carbohydrate
metabolism. PLP is also involved with lipid metabolism. Vitamin
B6 plays a role in immune function.

Healthy sources of vitamin B6 include:

- Banana
- Cereal grain (up to 25% of daily value)
- Carrots
- Chicken
- Spinach
- Legumes such as beans and lentils
- Peas
- Turkey
- Eggs
- Fish such as salmon
- Milk
- Orange juice

Vitamin B6 plays a role in the control of blood levels of
homocysteine. High levels of homocysteine increases the risk of
heart disease.

Daily Required Amount of Vitamin B6

The daily required amount of vitamin B6 is as follows:

Males 14 to 50 years of age require about 1.3 mg per day

Females 14 to 50 years of age requires about 1.2 mg per day

Males over 50 years old require about 1.6 mg per day

Females over 50 years old require about 1.5 mg per day

Vitamin B7 (Biotin)

Vitamin B7 is water soluble. It enhances the breakdown of carbohydrates, fat and proteins. This leads to the production of energy. The deficiency of vitamin B7 results in dermatitis and conjunctivitis. Biotin is also associated with alopecia or hair loss. Biotin from natural foods supports healthy skin, hair and nails.

Healthy sources of biotin include:

- Bananas
- Carrots
- Cauliflower
- Cereals
- Salmon

How about Biotin Shampoos for Hair Health?

The realization that biotin is beneficial for hair has given rise to a whole new breed of shampoos containing biotin. Biotin is not well absorbed through the skin so shampoos with added biotin are not very helpful for hair loss. So for your hair health, eat your way to healthier hair through biotin intake. Do not wash your way to weary hands with biotin shampoos; with barely any benefit. There is a big difference between ingested biotin and biotin applied to the skin.

Daily Required Amount of Vitamin B7

The daily required amount of vitamin B7 is as follows:

Teens and adults require about 35 mcg per day.
Pregnant females and nursing mothers require about 40 mcg per day.

Vitamin B9 (Folate, Folic Acid)

Vitamin B9 is water soluble. It plays a role in the breakdown of carbohydrates for the production of energy. It also enhances the breakdown of fat and proteins. It helps in the production of the genetic material of the body; the DNA (deoxyribonucleic acid) and RNA (ribonucleic acid). Folic acid is very important for pregnant women.

Deficiency of vitamin B9 is associated with anemia. Folate is available in natural foods. Folate from food is converted into folic acid in the body and absorbed. So folic acid is the utilizable form of folate in the body. It helps to prevent anemia. It enhances healthy skin and hair.

Healthy sources of vitamin B9 include:

- Green leafy vegetables such as spinach
- Asparagus
- Broccoli
- Fish such as salmon
- Legumes such as beans
- Orange juice
- Pumpkin seeds
- Sunflower seeds
- Strawberry
- Bran cereal

Dark green leafy spinach contains up to 20 % of the daily required amount of folate. Folate gets its name from the Latin word "folium" for leaf (2).

Folic Acid (Vitamin B9) and Cyanocobalamin (Vitamin B12)

It is very important for older adults to be aware of the relationship between folic acid and vitamin B_{12} because they are at greater risk of having a vitamin B_{12} deficiency (2). Folic acid can mask the symptoms of vitamin B12 deficiency. Unfortunately, folic acid will not correct changes in the nervous system that result from vitamin B_{12} deficiency. Permanent nerve damage can occur if vitamin B_{12} deficiency is not treated (2).

Is There Any Harm with Folate (Vitamin B9)?

When folate is taken naturally through the diet it causes no harm. It is a water soluble vitamin, so any excess intake is usually lost in the urine (2).

Daily Required Amount of Vitamin B9

The daily required amount of vitamin B9 is as follows:

Teens and adults require about 400 mcg per day
Pregnant women and nursing mothers require about 550 mcg

Vitamin B12 (Cyanocobalamin)

Vitamin B12 is water soluble. It is a vitamin that contains the metal ion known as cobalt. Vitamin B12 compounds are therefore referred to as Cobalamin. It enhances the formation of healthy red blood cells. It facilitates the maintenance of the central nervous system. Vitamin B12 is also believed to enhance cognitive function.

Deficiency of vitamin B12 can results in a number of problems. Deficiency causes megaloblastic anemia. Fatigue for no reason can be due to anemia. Deficiency in this vitamin also causes nerve problems. It also causes memory problems. Complication in health can be avoided by resolving vitamin B12 deficiency. There is a relationship between vitamin B12 and folic acid. When folic acid is taken in large quantity, it could mask vitamin B12 deficiency symptoms.

Healthy sources of vitamin B12 include:

- Fish
- Dairy products.
- Poultry
- Bran cereal

Vitamin B12 is only available in animal products. It can easily be obtained by people who drink milk and those who eat fortified cereals. Those who eat fish and poultry will also obtain the vitamin. Vegetarians can obtain vitamin B12 by eating fortified breakfast cereals. It is very important to treat vitamin B12 deficiency promptly. This is true in infants as well. Undetected and untreated vitamin B12 deficiency in infants can result in severe and permanent neurological damage (3).

It is critical for vegetarians to include foods with adequate vitamin B12 in their diet. This is the case because the Vegetarian diet supplies a lot of folate which can mask the symptoms of vitamin B12 deficiency and result in serious health problems.

Is There Any Harm with Vitamin B12?

Vitamin B12 is not one of those vitamins with concern about harm from consumption. Under normal circumstances vitamin B12 intake causes no harm.

Daily Required Amount of Vitamin B12

The amount of vitamin B12 you need each day depends on your age (3).

Average daily recommended amounts for different ages are listed below in micrograms (mcg) [3]:

Birth to 6 months	0.4 mcg
Infants 7–12 months	0.5 mcg
Children 1–3 years	0.9 mcg
Children 4–8 years	1.2 mcg
Children 9–13 years	1.8 mcg
Teens 14–18 years	2.4 mcg
Adults	2.4 mcg
Pregnant teens and women	2.6 mcg
Breastfeeding teens and women	2.8 mcg

Vitamin C (Ascorbic acid)

Vitamin C is water soluble. It is an antioxidant that helps to reduce the free radicals that cause damage in the body. It boosts the immune system. It is believed to function as an antihistamine. It enhances healthy skin, hair and nails. Vitamin C is also believed to minimize wrinkling of the skin by protecting it. Deficiency results in Scurvy.

Healthy sources of vitamin C include:

- Broccoli
- Blackberries
- Cherries
- Guava
- Grapefruits
- Kiwi fruit
- Lemons
- Limes
- Oranges
- Orange juice
- Strawberries
- Tangerines
- Tomatoes

Scurvy is fetal if it is not treated (4). People who get little or no vitamin C (below about 10 mg per day) for many weeks can get scurvy (4). Scurvy causes fatigue and the inflammation of the gums, small red or purple spots on the skin, joint pain, poor wound healing, and corkscrew hairs (4). Additional signs of scurvy include depression as well as swollen, bleeding gums and loosening or loss of teeth (4). People with scurvy can also develop anemia (4).

Reduction of free radicals by vitamin C is very beneficial to the body. Free radicals are compounds formed when our bodies convert the food we eat into energy (4). People are also exposed to free radicals in the environment from cigarette smoke, air pollution, and ultraviolet light from the sun (4). The body also needs vitamin C to make collagen a protein required to help wounds heal (4). In addition, vitamin C improves the absorption of iron from plant-based foods and helps the immune system work properly to protect the body from disease (4).

The vitamin C content of food may be reduced by prolonged storage and by cooking. Steaming or microwaving may lessen cooking losses (4). Fortunately, many of the best food sources of vitamin C, such as fruits and vegetables, are usually eaten raw (4).

Vitamin C deficiency is uncommon in developed countries but can still occur in people with limited food variety (5)

How about Taking Excess (Or Too Much) Vitamin C?

Obtaining vitamin C from natural sources is not likely to result in Vitamin C overdose. Overdose of vitamin C can occur if vitamin C supplement is taken in excess. Vitamin C does not have major problem with toxicity.

However, overdose of vitamin C could cause the following:

- Abdominal cramp
- Diarrhea
- Heart burn

Daily Required Amount of Vitamin C

The amount of vitamin C you need each day depends on your age (4). Average daily recommended amounts for different ages are listed below in milligrams (mg) [4].

Birth to 6 months	40 mg
Infants 7–12 months	50 mg
Children 1–3 years	15 mg
Children 4–8 years	25 mg
Children 9–13 years	45 mg
Teens 14–18 years (boys)	75 mg
Teens 14–18 years (girls)	65 mg
Adults (men)	90 mg
Adults (women)	75 mg
Pregnant teens	80 mg
Pregnant women	85 mg
Breastfeeding teens	115 mg
Breastfeeding women	120 mg

If you smoke, add 35 mg to the above values to calculate your total daily recommended amount (4).

Vitamin D (Cholecalciferol)

Vitamin D is fat soluble. It is needed for strong bones and teeth. Vitamin D enhances calcium absorption therefore it can help to protect from osteoporosis. Vitamin D deficiency results in rickets and osteomalacia (which are explained below).

The body produces Vitamin D. Being indoors all the time might interfere with vitamin D production and result in deficiency. Exposure to the sun is needed for the body to produce vitamin D. It is difficult to be vitamin D deficient with exposure to the sun and intake of vitamin D through the diet. Prolonged exposure to the sun is not necessary for vitamin D production. About 15 minutes of exposure to the sun is enough for vitamin D production.

Healthy sources of vitamin D include:

- Cheese
- Eggs yolk
- Fortified milk
- Yogurt
- Mushrooms (Dried Shitake)
- Bran cereal (fortified)
- Salmon

People who get little vitamin D may develop thin and brittle bones, a condition known as rickets in children and osteomalacia in adults (6). Vitamin D is important to the body in many other ways as well. Muscles need it to move, for example, nerves need it to carry messages between the brain and every body part, and the immune system needs vitamin D to fight off invading bacteria and viruses (6).

Initial symptoms of vitamin D deficiency can possibly be missed. Symptoms of bone pain and muscle weakness can indicate inadequate vitamin D levels, but such symptoms can be subtle and go undetected in the initial stages (7).

Is There Any Harm with Vitamin D?

There can be possible toxicity with vitamin D. Signs of toxicity include nausea, vomiting, poor appetite, constipation, weakness and weight loss (6). And by raising blood levels of calcium, too much vitamin D can cause confusion, disorientation and problems with heart rhythm (6). Excess vitamin D can also damage the kidneys (6).

Excessive sun exposure doesn't cause vitamin D poisoning because the body limits the amount of this vitamin it produces (6). Excessive exposure to the sun can harm the skin in some ways. Skin cancers can develop in some people due to excessive exposure to the sun. If you are going to be exposed excessively to the sun or for a prolonged period of time, protect your skin. Apply sunscreen to your skin with SPF value of 30.

Daily Required Amount of Vitamin D

The amount of vitamin D you need each day depends on your age (6). Average daily recommended amounts from the Food and Nutrition Board (a national group of experts) for different ages are listed below in International Units (IU) [6]:

Birth to 12 months	400 IU
Children 1–13 years	600 IU
Teens 14–18 years	600 IU
Adults 19–70 years	600 IU
Adults 71 years and older	800 IU
Pregnant and breastfeeding women	600 IU

Conversion of Vitamin D Daily Amount from IU to Mcg

40 IU of vitamin D is equivalent to 1 mcg

400 IU of vitamin D is equivalent to 10 mcg

600 IU of vitamin D is equivalent to 15 mcg

800 IU of vitamin D is equivalent to 20 mcg

Vitamin E (Tocopherols)

Vitamin E is fat soluble. As a fat soluble vitamin, it needs fat for its absorption and any condition that make people unable to absorb fat can make them deficient in vitamin E. It is an antioxidant that works against destructive free radicals that cause diseases. It promotes healthy skin. It enhances the formation of red blood cells. It is helpful in the maintenance of healthy blood vessels. It enhances the maintenance of the central nervous system. Deficiency of vitamin E results in hemolytic anemia in new born.

Healthy sources of vitamin E include:

- Avocado
- Broccoli
- Green leafy vegetables such as spinach
- Kiwi fruit
- Mango
- Nuts such as almonds and walnuts
- Sunflower seeds
- Some cereals
- Tomato (Raw)

The body also needs vitamin E to boost its immune system so that it can fight off invading bacteria and viruses (8). It helps to widen blood vessels and keep blood from clotting within them (8). In addition, cells use vitamin E to interact with each other and to carry out many important functions (8).

Many claims have been made about vitamin E's potential to promote health and prevent and treat disease (9). The mechanisms by which vitamin E might provide this protection include its function as an antioxidant and its roles in anti-inflammatory processes, inhibition of platelet aggregation, and immune enhancement (9).

Obtaining Daily Required Amount of Vitamin E

Vitamin E is one of those vitamins that you need conscious efforts to ensure that you are getting enough of it, every day in your foods. Unlike some vitamins such as vitamins A and C that are in a lot of foods, vitamin E is not in as many foods. Make efforts to include foods with vitamin E in your diet so that you will get enough vitamin E daily. It has numerous benefits. Include nuts and also some seeds in your diet. One serving of almonds which is about 24 nuts contains about one-third of the daily required amount of vitamin E. Also eat other foods such as broccoli daily as well as green spinach.

How about Taking Excess (Or Too Much) Vitamin E?

Obtaining vitamin E from natural sources such as foods is not likely to result in Vitamin E overdose. If excess amount of vitamin E supplement is taken, there could be problem with toxicity and harm. This is particularly bad for people who already have chronic medical conditions.

Daily Required Amount of Vitamin E

The amount of vitamin E you need each day depends on your age (8). Average daily recommended intakes are listed below in milligrams (mg) and in International Units (IU).

Package labels list the amount of vitamin E in foods and dietary supplements in IU [8].

Birth to 6 months	4 mg (6 IU)
Infants 7–12 months	5 mg (7.5 IU)
Children 1–3 years	6 mg (9 IU)
Children 4–8 years	7 mg (10.4 IU)
Children 9–13 years	11 mg (16.4 IU)
Teens 14–18 years	15 mg (22.4 IU)
Adults	15 mg (22.4 IU)
Pregnant teens and women	15 mg (22.4 IU)
Breastfeeding teens and women	19 mg (28.4 IU

Vitamin K (Phylloquinones)

Vitamin K is fat soluble. It helps with the production of protein for the clotting of the blood. Deficiency of vitamin K results in bleeding diathesis (predisposition to bleeding). Healthy sources include:

- Broccoli
- Dark green spinach
- Dark green lettuce
- Dark green collard green

People who are taking blood thinners such as warfarin or undergoing anticoagulation therapy need to be careful with vitamin K. Once stabilized on warfarin vitamin K intake needs to be consistent and not be altered. These people should avoid large amounts of green leafy vegetables. Too much vitamin K could decrease the thinning of the blood and blot clot could be formed. Anyone on a blood thinner should work with their doctor or pharmacist to ensure adequate monitoring. Usually for patients on warfarin, the International Normalized Ratio is measured frequently and the result is used to adjust the dose of warfarin to ensure safe optimal therapy.

Prothrombin Time (PT) and International Normalized Ratio (INR)

Prothrombin time (PT) is a blood test. It is usually measured in seconds. It is used to determine how long (in seconds) it takes for your blood to clot. INR is a ratio that is calculated using the result of prothrombin time tests.

Daily Required Amount of Vitamin K

Teens (male and females) require about 75 mcg per day
Males and females 19 years of age and older require 90 mcg per day

Supplements: Should I Take Vitamin Supplements?

Americans spend literarily millions of dollars on vitamin supplements every year. The use of vitamin supplements is so widespread that some people believe that it is required to be healthy. This mindset is the mega force that propels the popularity of vitamin supplements today.

I have to say that I almost joined the vitamin supplement movement. My family, however, decided that we will choose healthy foods and obtain our vitamins naturally. My husband, Dr. J. Okoli, did not want it any other way. We chose dietary vitamin sources in spite of our four very active children who were participating heavily in sports and other activities including; basketball, soccer, volleyball, figure skating, gymnastics, dance, cheer leading, music, piano and performing. In our home, good energy was never a problem.

In professional setting, I give counsel to patients on vitamin supplements but I also recommend healthy eating at every opportunity. To answer the question, "should I take vitamin supplements?" we need to consider a few things:

(1) Firstly, the primary recommended source for daily required vitamins is through natural healthy foods. Natural healthy foods if taken daily will easily supply you with the vitamins that you need. This will free you from the concern of

missing some doses of the vitamins that you need daily if you were to take supplements.

(2) Secondly, the vitamins in food will be easily absorbed and used by your body without any problems.

(3) Thirdly, you will not have the temptation to eat carelessly because you have taken some vitamin supplements. This may sound basic but it is very important. When you know that you need to obtain your daily vitamins from foods, this will motivate you to eat healthy foods as well as diversify what you eat. You will improve your overall health in the process.

(4) The dosage form of the vitamin supplements might be an issue and getting enough of each required vitamin from the dosage forms might be a problem also.

(5) Furthermore, healthy cereals are heavily fortified with the daily vitamins. They contain at least 10% of the daily value that is required for the vitamins. As a matter of fact, most of the cereals contain 25% of the daily value of most of the daily vitamins in one serving of the cereal. Milk and 100% natural juices are also fortified with vitamins.

(6) Wrong amounts or excessive intake of vitamins supplements can even be harmful to the body and result in toxicity. This is especially true of the fat soluble vitamins. For example, excessive intake of vitamin A supplement in the form of retinol can lead to the breakdown of bones. Obtaining vitamin A from plant based foods in the form of

beta- carotene does not cause the breakdown of bones. Harm or toxicity can also occur with too much vitamins D and E supplements.

(7) Finally, the purchase of the vitamins represents additional expense that you do not have to worry about if you eat healthy foods; especially if you have financial concerns. Even if you do not have financial concerns purchasing vitamin supplements can represent avoidable expense. Your time is saved as well.

So my recommendation is to commit to healthy eating and not worry about supplementation. Healthy natural foods are superior vitamin sources and are more than able to supply your body with the daily vitamins that is required for various functions.

Taking Vitamin Supplements: Any Exceptions?

Yes, there are few cases where vitamin supplementation is mandatory. Such cases include:

(1) Pregnancy

Every pregnant woman in addition to eating healthy foods should be on prenatal vitamins so that the baby will be supplied with all that it needs to grow and develop without defects.

(2) Diagnosed vitamin deficiency

Anyone who is diagnosed with vitamin deficiency needs to take vitamin supplements until the deficiency is resolved. After the resolution of the deficiency, healthy foods need to be used to maintain good health and avoid future deficiency.

Action Summary # 11

Strive to obtain your vitamins from your diet; through the consumption of healthy, fresh, natural, and whole foods. Enjoy the beneficial function of vitamins in helping to remove toxins from the body. Some are also available from fish, poultry, dairy and fortified cereals.

In some situations some people may be deficient in certain vitamins. Resolution of the vitamin deficiency can be accomplished. Avoid depending on vitamins supplements.

Chapter Twelve

Minerals

Minerals are also used by the body in various processes that enhance the maintenance of the body. While calcium is abundant in the body, a lot of minerals are used in small amounts by the body. Like vitamins, minerals can also be obtained from fresh healthy foods. A lot of foods are fortified with minerals. Package labels display the minerals with which certain foods are fortified.

Calcium

Calcium is the most abundant mineral in the body. It is very important in the maintenance of healthy bones. It is also very useful in the maintenance of the structure of the teeth. Most of the calcium in the body is stored in the bone. Some calcium is also stored in the teeth. Vitamin D improves the absorption of calcium.

The body also needs calcium for muscles to move and for nerves to carry messages between the brain and every body part (10). In addition, calcium is used to help blood vessels move blood throughout the body and to help release hormones and enzymes that affect almost every function in the human body (10).

Insufficient intakes of calcium do not produce obvious symptoms in the short term because the body maintains calcium levels in the blood by taking it from bone (10). Over the long term, intakes of calcium below recommended levels have health consequences, such as causing low bone mass (osteopenia) and increasing the risks of osteoporosis and bone fractures (10). Osteoporosis is the thinning and weakening of the tissues of the bone. Bone pain is a symptom of osteoporosis.

Symptoms of serious calcium deficiency include numbness and tingling in the fingers, convulsions, and abnormal heart rhythms that can lead to death if not corrected (10). These symptoms occur almost always in people with serious health problems or who are undergoing certain medical treatments (10).

Calcium can be obtained from some healthy foods. Some beverages are fortified with calcium, including 100% juices. Calcium sources include:

- Broccoli
- Blackberries
- Low fat milk
- Low fat yogurt
- Low fat cheese
- Nuts such as almonds
- Orange juice with calcium
- Pink salmon
- Dark green spinach
- Turnip greens
- Tofu

How about Taking Excess (Or Too Much) Calcium?

Obtaining too much calcium from the diet is unlikely. Too much calcium can be obtained through calcium supplementation. Getting too much calcium can cause constipation (10). It might also interfere with the body's ability to absorb iron and zinc, but this effect is not well established (10). In adults, too much calcium (from dietary supplements but not food) might increase the risk of kidney stones (10).

Daily Required Amount of Calcium

The amount of calcium you need each day depends on your age (10). Average daily recommended amounts are listed below in milligrams (mg) [10]:

Birth to 6 months	200 mg
Infants 7–12 months	260 mg
Children 1–3 years	700 mg
Children 4–8 years	1,000 mg
Children 9–13 years	1,300 mg
Teens 14–18 years	1,300 mg
Adults 19–50 years	1,000 mg
Adult men 51–70 years	1,000 mg
Adult women 51–70 years	1,200 mg
Adults 71 years and older	1,200 mg
Pregnant and breastfeeding teens	1,300 mg

Pregnant and breastfeeding adults	1,000 mg

Iron and Other Trace Minerals

Trace Minerals

Trace minerals are those minerals which are required in small amounts by the body. They include iron. They also include chromium, copper, iodine, magnesium, selenium, and zinc. The best way to obtain these trace elements is by eating a variety of fresh healthy foods.

Iron

Iron is an essential mineral that is used by the body. Most of the iron in the body is in the red blood cells. It is involved with carrying oxygen to the tissues. Having adequate iron in the body boosts energy. Deficiency in iron results in anemia. As a result of the decrease in iron, the amount of oxygen that is delivered to the tissues decreases. This will result in tiredness or fatigue. Iron can be obtained from the diet.

Healthy sources of iron include:

- Blackberries
- Black eyed peas
- Chicken
- Fish

- Lentils
- Nuts such as almonds
- Green leafy vegetables such as spinach
- Tofu
- Oatmeal (100% whole grain)
- Seeds such as pumpkin seeds
- Turkey

Iron from lean beef is most easily absorbed.

Iron Supplements

Iron supplements may be needed by people in some situations. People who will need Iron supplements include;

- Pregnant women
- People who are diagnosed with iron deficiency anemia
- Teenage girls who have reason to be anemic

If iron supplement is indicated for you, take it with food to minimize side effects, but do not take it with milk. It is important to remember that iron supplements can be constipating. Make every effort to eat a lot of fruits (including whole oranges) and plenty of vegetables (including broccoli and spinach) while you are taking iron supplements. Eat oatmeal from 100% whole grain source with the supplement. Take one cup of orange juice a day with it. Also take plenty of water, up to three liters a day. If you still feel constipated, take over the counter stool softener with the iron.

My recommendation for a stool softener is docusate sodium. This is usually gentle. Its laxative effect is experienced in one full day (24 hours) or two days. Full effect could take three to four days for some people. Avoid taking it long term. It is recommended that you do not take it for more than seven days unless directed to do otherwise by your physician. Take it only when you have to. If you use it long term, its effectiveness might be diminished. Docusate sodium does not diminish nutrient absorption from the gastrointestinal tract.

Medication should be the last resort for pregnant women. The above dietary measures with lots of fiber and lots of water as well as daily walk should be very helpful. It is used in pregnancy if lifestyle modifications prove inadequate for constipation relief. Check with your doctor before using docusate sodium if you are pregnant.

Some people can get diarrhea with iron supplement. Note any side effects that you may have with it and report bothersome side effects to your doctor. If you have any skin rash or facial swelling while on the supplement, stop taking it and report those promptly to your physician.

When iron deficiency is diagnosed, the deficiency usually can be rectified once iron supplementation is initiated and adhered to. Iron deficiency is usually monitored until it is rectified.

Physicians monitor the effectiveness of iron supplements by measuring laboratory indices, including reticulocyte count (levels of newly formed red blood cells), hemoglobin levels, and ferritin levels (11). Hemoglobin is a red blood cell protein. It carries oxygen to the tissues and organs and also carries carbon dioxide from the tissues and organs back to the lungs. Ferritin is a blood cell protein that contains iron.

In the presence of anemia, reticulocyte counts will begin to rise after a few days of supplementation. Hemoglobin usually increases within 2 to 3 weeks of starting iron supplementation (11).

There are many causes of anemia, including iron deficiency (11). This means that someone can be anemic without necessarily being iron deficient. The cause of anemia can be determined by the physician. After a thorough evaluation, physicians can diagnose the cause of anemia and prescribe the appropriate treatment (11).

How about Taking Excess (Or Too Much) Iron?

There is considerable potential for iron toxicity because very little iron is excreted from the body (11). Thus, iron can accumulate in body tissues and organs when normal storage sites are full (11). Hemochromatosis is a condition where the body absorbs too much iron and stores them in various organs, which can eventually lead to diseases. Example, people with hemochromatosis are at risk of developing iron toxicity because of their high iron stores (11).

Daily Required Amount of Iron

About 10 mg per day for males 14 to 50 years of age
About 16 mg per day for females 14 to 50 years of age
About 28 mg per day for pregnant females
About 8 milligrams for males and females over 50 years of age

People who engage in intense exercise should ensure that they have adequate iron. Some people experience shortness of breath during exercise due to iron deficiency.

If you are not sure that you have sufficient iron, talk to your doctor. Your doctor can help determine if you have sufficient iron.

Elemental Iron

Note the amount of elemental iron in the supplement that you are buying; if your physician recommends iron supplement for you. Elemental iron which is listed on the package label of iron supplements represents the amount of iron in the supplement that is available for absorption. Different forms of iron supplements contain different amounts of elemental iron. Take the amount of iron that is recommended for you per day to help resolve your deficiency.

Other Trace Minerals

Chromium

Chromium is one of the trace minerals that are needed by the body. It is involved in metabolism. It is also involved with the appropriate use of glucose. Healthy sources of chromium include broccoli.

How about Taking Excess (Or Too Much) Chromium

There are not many side effects that are associated with the intake of chromium.

Adequate Intake of Chromium

For teens and adults adequate intake of chromium is about 30 to 35 mcg per day.

Copper

Copper is one of the trace minerals that the body needs. It is involved in making red blood cells and enhances healthy bones. Deficiency of copper could enhance anemia and osteoporosis.

Healthy sources of copper include:

- Avocados
- Bran cereals
- Dark green leafy vegetables
- Mushroom

- Nuts such as almonds

How about Taking Excess (Or Too Much) Copper

There is toxicity with excess copper. In excess it gets deposited in organs and lead to problems or disorders.

Daily Intake of Copper

Daily intake recommended for teens and adults is about 900 mcg per day.

Iodine

Iodine is one of the trace minerals which the body uses. The body needs iodine to make thyroid hormones. These hormones control the body's metabolism and many other important functions (12). The body also needs thyroid hormones for proper bone and brain development during pregnancy and infancy (12). Getting enough iodine is important for everyone, especially infant and women who are pregnant (12).

Healthy sources of iodine include:

- Iodized salt
- Shrimp
- Milk
- Yogurt

Adequate iodine intake is critical. Eating shrimps about twice a week and also using iodized salt about twice a week and eating low-fat or non-fat yogurt several times a week along with low fat milk should supply adequate iodine. One serving of iodized salt (one-fourth teaspoonful) contains about 45 % of the daily required iodine.

People who don't get enough iodine cannot make sufficient amounts of thyroid hormone (12). This can cause many problems. In pregnant women, severe iodine deficiency can permanently harm the fetus by causing stunted growth, mental retardation, and delayed sexual development (12). Less severe iodine deficiency can cause lower-than-average IQ in infants and children and decrease adults' ability to work and think clearly (12).

How about Taking Excess (Or Too Much) Iodine?

Taking excess amount of iodine can cause a health problem. Too much iodine would result in a condition known as goiter (which is enlarged thyroid gland). This enlarged thyroid gland can be visible. High iodine intakes can also cause thyroid gland inflammation and thyroid cancer (12). Getting a very large dose of iodine (several grams, for example) can cause burning of the mouth, throat, and stomach; fever; stomach pain; nausea; vomiting; diarrhea; weak pulse; and coma (12).

Daily Required Amount of Iodine

The amount of iodine you need each day depends on your age (12).

Average daily recommended amounts are listed below in micrograms (mcg) [12].

Birth to 6 months	110 mcg
Infants 7–12 months	130 mcg
Children 1–8 years	90 mcg
Children 9–13 years	120 mcg
Teens 14–18 years	150 mcg
Adults	150 mcg
Pregnant teens and women	220 mcg
Breastfeeding teens and women	290 mcg

Magnesium

Magnesium is one of the more abundant minerals in the body. It is found in bone and other parts of the body. Magnesium deficiency can result in weakness. Having deficiency of this mineral can eventually lead to low calcium (hypocalcemia).

Healthy sources of magnesium include:

- Bran cereal
- Nuts such as almonds

- Spinach
- Pumpkin seeds

Eating a variety of whole grains, legumes, and vegetables (especially dark-green, leafy vegetables) every day will help provide recommended intakes of magnesium and maintain normal storage levels of this mineral (13). Increasing dietary intake of magnesium can often restore mildly depleted magnesium levels (13). However, increasing dietary intake of magnesium may not be enough to restore very low magnesium levels to normal (13). If you have very low magnesium, your doctor can work with you to correct deficiency.

How about Taking Excess (Or Too Much) Magnesium?

It is unlikely to get too much magnesium from diet. Too much magnesium can be taken through supplement. Too much magnesium can cause symptoms that include muscle weakness and difficulty with breathing.

Daily Required Amount of Magnesium

The daily required amount of magnesium is as follows:

Males 15 to 18 years of age requires about 410 mg per day
Females 15 to 18 years old requires about 560 mg per day

Males 19 to 30 years old requires about 400 mg per day
Females 19 to 30 years old requires about 310 mg per day

Males over 30 years of age requires about 420 mg per day

Females over 30 years old requires about 320 mg per day

Selenium

Selenium is one of the trace minerals that the body needs. It is used in making certain enzymes which are needed for body functions including antioxidant functions.

How about Taking Excess (Or Too Much) Selenium

Excess selenium intake from diet is not very common. Selenium toxicity can occur with symptoms that include stomach upset and fatigue.

Daily Required Amount of Selenium

Teens and adults require about 50 to 60mcg per day

Zinc

Zinc is one of the trace minerals. The body needs it in small amount. Zinc is found in cells throughout the body (14). It helps the immune system fight off invading bacteria and viruses (14). The body also needs zinc to make proteins and DNA, the genetic material in all cells. During pregnancy, infancy, and childhood, the body needs zinc to grow and develop properly (14). Zinc also helps wounds heal and is important for proper senses of taste and smell (14). Zinc is believed to facilitate the recovery from common cold.

Zinc deficiency can result in a number of health problems. It causes slow growth in infants and children, delayed sexual development in adolescents and impotence in men (14). Zinc deficiency also causes hair loss, diarrhea, eye and skin sores and loss of appetite (14). Weight loss, problems with wound healing, decreased ability to taste food, and lower alertness levels can also occur (14). If you experience any of these symptoms, let your doctor help you determine if you have zinc deficiency.

Healthy sources of zinc include:

- Fortified cereals
- Almonds and some of the other nuts
- Beans
- Lean red meat
- Lobster and oyster
- Pumpkin seeds

Vegetarians can also increase their zinc intake by consuming more leavened grain products (such as bread) than unleavened products (such as crackers) because leavening partially breaks down the phytate; thus, the body absorbs more zinc from leavened grains than unleavened grains (15). Vegetarians need higher intake of zinc than is recommended because the grains and beans that they eat decrease zinc absorption by the body.

How about Taking Excess (Or Too Much) Zinc?

There can be a problem with taking excess or too much zinc. Signs of too much zinc include nausea, vomiting, loss of appetite, stomach cramps, diarrhea, and headaches (14). When people take too much zinc for a long time, they sometimes have problems such as low copper levels, lower immunity, and low levels of HDL cholesterol (the "good" cholesterol) (14).

Daily Required Amount of Zinc

The amount of zinc you need each day depends on your age (14). Average daily recommended
amounts for different ages are listed below in milligrams (mg) [14]:

Birth to 6 months	2 mg
Infants 7–12 months	3 mg
Children 1–3 years	3 mg
Children 4–8 years	5 mg
Children 9–13 years	8 mg
Teens 14–18 years (boys)	11 mg
Teens 14–18 years (girls)	9 mg
Adults (men)	11 mg
Adults (women)	8 mg
Pregnant teens	12 mg
Pregnant women	11 mg

Breastfeeding teens	13 mg
Breastfeeding women	12 mg

Action Summary # 12

Endeavor to obtain your minerals through fresh healthy foods and fortified foods. Iron supplementation might be needed in some cases. Your physician will advice you on any deficiencies and how best to replenish them.

Chapter Thirteen

Healthy Choices and Actions

Good health and wellbeing are the result of a combination of healthy choices and actions. These work together in many ways to keep you healthy, energetic, and fully functional. Isolated healthy action such as right food without exercise or exercise without the right food is not sufficient for you to be healthy. As seen in previous chapters, good health is enhanced by the following:

(a) Eating healthy recommended foods

(b) Exercising regularly

(c) Getting good rest regularly or frequently

(d) Making good healthy choices that enhance your health

Eating Healthy Recommended Foods

How about People Who Eat What They Want and Take Chances with Health?

When it comes to healthy living, there are two groups of people. Those who would hold onto a healthy lifestyle and those who are either not interested in it or are partially committed to it. Some in the later group will say, "I simply do not like eating healthy, I will take my chances and eat what I enjoy." This is a dangerous stand to take. Health should never be left to chance or one will be forced to choose from difficult unfortunate options.

The functions of the body are not affected by food taste. They are affected by the nutrient quality of the food that you eat. The body functions optimally with the right nutrients and actions; and malfunctions with the wrong nutrients and actions. Battling preventable illness that can slow you down in every way is not a favorable option. Good health, on the other hand, empowers you to enjoy the most out of your life.

I believe that good taste is important, so I find good tasting healthy alternatives to unhealthy foods so that I can maintain a healthy lifestyle. For some people, it will take some time to get used to eating differently for good health. If you start eating healthier, after sometime you will get used to your new eating habit and begin to feel good about it. Your body will also feel and look good for it. It is like people whose country change from left hand drive to right hand drive on the road. Some people believe that they will never get used to driving on the right side of the road after driving on the left side for so many years. These people drive on the right side anyway, because it is the law. After some years, they get so used to driving on the right side that it comes naturally. Changing to healthy eating from unhealthy eating is the same way. Once you get started and stay consistent, it will become part of your daily life and the benefits part of your delight.

As healthy foods are eaten, healthy weight is not only achieved it is also maintained without difficulty. You will increase your chance of living a healthier and longer life.

Exercising Regularly

The benefits of exercise are obvious. Exercise increases high density lipoprotein (HDL) or good cholesterol. As HDL increases low density lipoprotein (LDL) or bad cholesterol decreases. HDL and LDL have inverse relationship. When your LDL decreases you will have less chance of having clogged arteries and your risk of various diseases decrease. Your will not be sluggish or easily out of breath with regular exercise.

Getting Good Sleep Regularly or Frequently

Your body performs some critical functions at night when you rest and sleep. Sufficient sleep is essential for optimal functioning of your immune system. You will be unable to stay healthy for a long time without good night sleep. If you eat the right foods, exercise regularly and not get sufficient rest, you could still be unhealthy. Adhere to good sleeping hygiene to facilitate good sleep and enjoy better health.

Making Good Healthy Choices that Enhance Your Health

To help consolidate healthy choices ponder the following seven questions:

(1) What actions do I need to take daily to achieve a healthy lifestyle?
(2) What can I add or remove from my diet to maintain good health and good weight?

(3) What has helped or hurt my chances of achieving my ideal weight?

(4) If I continue all that I am doing daily will I be healthy five years from now?

(5) Do I have good energy?

(6) Can I recommend what I am doing about my health with confidence to someone else and expect good result?

(7) Am I doing all that I can do to be healthy or have I given up on trying to be healthy?

Remember, when it comes to your health, a small change in lifestyle can have a big impact on your overall health. Switching to fresh foods and high fiber foods from processed foods, for instance, is one of those changes that can dramatically lower your risk of a host of diseases.

There is no one who cannot succeed in living a healthy lifestyle. In a matter of a few weeks, persistent healthy choices will yield result in better health, better feeling, and better looks. If you think right about your health, you will act right about your health. The biggest effort towards good health is in the thought. I cannot emphasize right thoughts enough. Right thinking effortlessly yields right actions. When it comes to health, consistent right actions will yield multiple health benefits that are desirable.

A Healthy Choice Deception

Some people are careful to count calories throughout the day to ensure that they are eating the right amount of calories per day. Some of these people include for their daily consumption foods that are very bad for them in spite of fitting into their calculated calories limit per day.

Is Counting Calories the Answer?

Some people over simplify healthy eating and say, "It is all about counting your calories." Healthy eating goes far beyond counting calories. All calories are not equal. Choosing inappropriate food and counting its calories is like getting on the wrong road to a desired destination and counting the mileage covered on the wrong road. Covering the required mileage for your destination on the wrong road cannot get you to your desired destination. We all know that it is important to be on the right road to a desired destination first before counting the mileage covered towards the desired destination. In the same way, it is important to choose the right food first before counting the calories in the food.

Calorie content alone is not adequate consideration in making food and snack choices. If you want a snack with 85 calories for instance, you could grab a medium sized apple or some sugar cookies or some candies. The cookies and candies in spite of matching the calories in the apple could increase your weight and diminish your health if you continue to eat them over time. Eating a medium sized apple will provide for you, in addition to the calories, about 4.3 grams of the fiber which your body needs. Candies and sugar cookies usually provide no fiber. The apple will also provide naturally vitamin A, vitamin B9, vitamin C, calcium, iron, potassium, and phosphorus that your body needs for better health. The sugar cookies and candies will result in rapid increase in your blood glucose levels which is not good for you. The apple does not have a high glycemic index so it will not result in a spike in your blood glucose level. The apple, because of the fiber that it contains, keeps you fuller and so you eat less. The sugar cookies or candies, on the other hand, could keep you less full and allow you to eat more as well as gain weight. Calorie content consideration is only helpful if the food is from a healthy source. Food and snack sources are critical for good health.

Benefits of Healthy Choices: Right Foods, Exercise, and Rest

Healthy choices made towards healthy living allow you to enjoy a lot of benefits including:

(1) Healthy weight

(2) Healthy skin

(3) Healthy hair and nails

(4) Good health

(5) Good energy

(6) Younger look

(7) Healthier long term vision

(8) Healthier mind

(9) Enhanced Immune system

(10)   Reduced stress and Good sleep

(11)   Avoidance of Obesity Surgery

Healthy Weight

Imagine Losing Weight without Even Thinking about It; the Best Weight Loss Strategy

Is it even possible to lose weight without stressing about it? Absolutely, you can lose weight while going about your daily life without focusing on it. You just focus on the right thoughts, the right foods, and the right actions and your weight will follow suit and change in the right direction. It will decreases consistently over time to a healthy range. This is the best weight loss strategy.

Healthy Skin

Some of the toxic, fatty, and processed foods that people eat even cause the skin to break out. A high-fat diet is also believed to speed-up the aging of the skin. The right nutrients that combat free radicals slow down the aging process. This is beneficial to the skin. Some fresh foods and fish like salmon and proper hydration enhance skin health and appearance.

Healthy Hair

Healthy eating also enhances healthy hair. The B vitamins are essential for the maintenance of healthy hair. The B vitamins include; Vitamin B1 (Thiamine), Vitamin B6 (Pyridoxine), Vitamin B7 (Biotin), Vitamin B9 (Folic acid) and Vitamin B12 (Cobalamin).

Sources of the B vitamins include:

- Apples
- Bananas
- Chili (hot) peppers
- 100 % orange juice
- Spinach
- Bran cereal

Vitamin B7 (Biotin) is worth noting in this area. It is believed that biotin from natural foods enhances the health of the skin, hair, and nails.

Natural food sources of biotin include:

- Avocado
- Bananas
- Carrots
- Cauliflower
- Certain cereals
- Grapefruit

- Nuts
- Salmon (especially if grilled)

Good Health

Healthy lifestyle yields good health. Exercising your muscles, for instance, increases their ability to use insulin and absorb glucose. This, in turn, keeps you healthier.

Good Energy

Good energy comes with healthy living. Healthy eating, for instance, decreases your disease risk. This minimizes your chance of being slowed down by possible damage to the body or disease symptoms. Healthy living also increases your energy in many other ways.

Younger Look

People do a lot of things these days to help them look young. Some, unfortunately, run into cosmetic mishap in the process and end up looking worse than they started. This happens in spite of all the efforts that they have put into the process and the pain they had to endure.

You can strive to look young from the inside to the outside. Healthy living rejuvenates your body. It allows you to enjoy a youthful appearance the natural way. You will have less damage inside your body and look younger and fresh on the outside.

Healthier Long Term Vision

We know that Vitamin A in carrots is good for our eyes and enhances vision. This includes night vision. Right fresh foods help people to maintain healthier vision as they get older and also help to protect against damage; as well as decrease degeneration of the eye.

Healthier Mind

Part of the benefit of choosing a healthy lifestyle is having a healthy mind. Healthy foods, adequate rest, and right thoughts can enhance your mental state and improve your memory. You will be refreshed emotionally.

Enhanced Immune System

Eating recommended foods and getting adequate sleep every day boosts the immune system. When the immune system is functioning properly, it protects the body against different kinds of infections including cold and flu (influenza).

Reduced Stress and Good Sleep

Combining healthy eating and regular exercise with good sleeping hygiene will greatly increase your chances of getting the sleep that your body needs daily. Sleep deprivation causes mental, emotional, and physical fatigue. Sleep deprivation also causes irritability. If it is prolonged, it can affect the ability of the body to function optimally daily. Enough sleep is beneficial in combating stress.

Obesity Surgery (Bariatric Surgery)

If unchecked, weight that increases rapidly and steadily over time results in obesity. When obesity becomes severe, or when excess weight is complicated by some disease states, bariatric surgery becomes a critical option for relief. I know some people who have weight issues addressed in this way. The most common bariatric surgery is gastric bypass. If any type of bariatric surgery is indicated, it is very important that a healthy lifestyle is adopted and adhered to following bariatric surgery. This includes appropriate nutrition. The recommended diet following surgery must be adhered to strictly to avoid problems or even repeat surgery.

The availability of bariatric surgery need not be an encouragement for an unhealthy lifestyle. Bariatric procedures are major operations with significant risks.

Avoidance of Obesity Surgery

Adhering to the guidelines of a healthy lifestyle as discussed in this book can help people to avoid obesity surgery and possible morbidity and mortality associated with it. This is crucial.

Healthy Choices for Seniors

Healthy living, which includes adequate rest, facilitates wellbeing for all seniors. It is also important that they proactively engage their minds profitably. Activities that prevent sedentary lifestyle need to be adopted and adhered to for better health.

Seniors who are taking multiple medications should consider using pill organizers to simplify taking daily medications. There are various options to choose from. It ranges from daily organizers to 30-day pill organizers. This is critical where people confuse the medications. It will help the right drug to be taken. Exception to this will be drugs that have to be dispensed in specific type of containers.

Healthy Choices for Athletes: From Professionals Down to Beginners

It is great to be gifted athletically. I played high school basketball for some years. I also had the opportunity to attend figure skating tests and competitions, gymnastics training and competitions up to Level 10, soccer and volleyball games, track and field meets, as well as numerous division I basketball games of my children sometimes in three states in one season. I have seen my children and the children of friends go from college sports to professional schools and national professional sports' leagues. Some professional athletes combine their very busy career with pursuit of advanced degree programs. I obtained a degree in Biochemistry as a young adult. I also obtained my doctor of pharmacy degree married to a busy husband with four children in sports and a hectic schedule. From my experience and observation, tremendous discipline is required to accomplish these tasks.

Most athletes already understand the role that hard work plays in their athletic success. The area that seem unclear to some athletes, however, is the importance of the other side of who they are. To have a full and balanced life, as well as maintain good mental health long term, every athlete should strive to be fully prepared physically and fully equipped mentally. To do this, the following are critical:

(1) Staying focused

(2) Avoiding poor academic and social choices

(3) Planning relaxation around healthy social activities

(4) Trusting in a higher power beyond yourself

(5) Developing your other skills

(6) Preparing for the next phase of life

(7) Enjoy contribution more than praise

Staying Focused

There are a lot of distractions that can negatively affect the focus of an athlete at every level. Discipline opened the door of athletics to you. Continue the good work that you started. Hard work is the only thing that you have full control of; allow it to work in your favor. Avoid falling prey to the discouragement that can come when you are denied recognition that is due to you. This is true no matter what happens. This mindset will give you confidence and ultimately work in your favor in your future life.

Your life has a broader scope than athletics. This type of confidence under pressure does not come naturally. It comes from determining to think ahead and not be caught up in the moment. Think beyond the big game or competition that went so wrong in spite of your great expectation. Your time to celebrate will eventually come even if it does not come this day.

Do not allow negative emotions to flourish in your mind. Continuous negative emotions are not good for your mental health. They could make you too unhealthy to enjoy yourself even when your time to shine in one area or another arrives. Emotional support is critical. Every athlete needs support especially as some important issues are out of their control. Make sure that you have people who support and encourage you.

I will mention briefly real life experiences of two athletes. These two athletes were much sought after in their sport. They happened to be in a group sport. For some reason they did not get as much opportunity to play in their sport as was expected. They did not get the recognition they were capable of as a consequence. One of them got so discouraged month after month and eventually got depressed. This discouragement and inability to stay positive caused a lot of emotional pain for the athlete and adversely affected important relationships.

The second athlete decided to pour the frustration of not playing into exceptional hard work and preparedness. This led to academic and athletic excellence as well as good opportunities. Furthermore, this athlete took advantage of encouragement. Some encouragers read the Bible to this athlete while others prayed. Emotional pain was minimized as a result.

It is vital to stay focused and maintain the hard work that athletes are capable of. This will open doors for you sooner or later. You will have plenty of opportunities to be celebrated, stand tall and hang onto hope for that day ahead.

Avoid Poor Choices and Adhere to Good Choices

Some athletes that I have known since my family got involved with sports make wrong choices that adversely affect their otherwise bright athletic future. Endeavor to make profitable choices. Poor choices include going to questionable places that will expose you to harm or trouble. Know the associations that you need to avoid. Avoid friends that will drag you down and slow down your progress. Surround yourself with people who make you better. Avoid the temptation of thinking that making poor social choices outside the gym or field does not matter as long as you continue to perform. Poor choices yield regrettable results sooner or later.

If you are a student, avoid skipping classes whether it can be overlooked or not. I know someone who lost a chance to be in the big league by doing that. Obtain promptly missed work when you cannot possibly be in class. Avoid settling for the minimum grades needed to continue with sports. Use available help if you need it to maximize grade. Avoid skipping study sessions that are provided for you.

If you do not have enough time to study, dictate your notes into an audio recorder. You can also record your classes if that is possible. Play back the class notes repeatedly on the way back from trips whether the trip went well or not. If the competition does not go well, correct mistakes where applicable and also prepare for good grades and enjoy the satisfaction that they bring. For courses that involve calculations record the formulae with explanations and play it repeatedly to enhance the mastering of the formulae. This will make your studying easier even with limited time. It will also make "A" grades possible. Aim at high grades.

Plan Relaxation around Healthy Social Activities

Watch events that are outside of your area of expertise. Explore and enjoy nature as much as possible. Get massage when possible. Do something that is clean, fun, and relaxing. Volunteer some of the time to help people who are not as fortunate as you are and enjoy the good feeling that go with such worthwhile activities.

Trust in a Higher Power beyond Yourself

When you have done all you know how to do to solve a problem but are unsuccessful, get help to find a good resolution for it. Even if you have done all you can and yet cannot help the situation, do not allow yourself to sink into despair. There must be other people who found solution for problems that are similar to yours. Some people trust the power of God to help them when they cannot help themselves. Some people insist on finding answers through prayers.

Develop Your Other Skills

Being able to continue in sports is wonderful but no one can be an athlete forever. Make every effort to develop skills that you can use after athletics. This will make things easier for you in the future.

Preparing for the Next Phase of Life

It is critical to prepare for the phase of your life after athletics or competitions. If you are a student, make sure that you obtain your degree. Insist on finishing what you started. If you are a professional athlete, seek out a way to prepare yourself for that stage of life that you will be facing at some point. Do this early in professional sports. Train for skills that will be immediately usable following retirement from professional sports. It applies whether competitions end from age or prematurely due to injury. Any athlete that focuses only on athletics is, unfortunately, doing himself or herself a disfavor. Preparing for the next level of your life cannot be overemphasized. This is applicable to athletic competitions from middle school to the professional level. If this is not done, unbearable mental stress that jeopardizes mental health can result.

After having sports in the center of one's life for so long, letting it go can be difficult. When the career in athletics ends, former athlete can feel lost, become overwhelmed, or even become depressed. Income could even become an issue for former professional athletes. Some athletes in spite of admirable income in athletics have even become bankrupt after professional sports. This reversal in fortune may negatively impact mental health. Being prepared ahead of time is the answer for a smooth and stress-free transition from professional athletic career to life after athletics.

Enjoy Contribution More Than Praise

This may seem basic but it is important. As you perform, learn to enjoy the contribution that you are making more than the praise that you are receiving. This is because if you focus on the praise, it might lead to exaggerated ego. Some people develop significant ego that end up hurting them and their relationships. This is true of people who have succeeded in various areas of life as well, including graduates of professional schools. Focusing on your contribution will help you enjoy making a difference. Focusing on your contribution will also help to protect you from crumbling when the praise is denied for any reason.

A Winning Edge

Some athletes have prepared themselves to win in game competitions and life competition beyond the games. They have been successful in meeting the two important objectives of hard work in sports and the development of usable skills after athletics. Those that have met these two goals include athletes who have proceeded to professional schools at the end of their athletic career or obtained a graduate degree on a part time basis as professional athletes. A third group obtained certificates in one form of fitness training or another and started businesses following their athletic career. A fourth group transitioned into other stable careers.

If athletes are prepared for life after athletics, this will help to reduce bothersome uncertainties that could accompany the completion of an athletic career. Proper planning ensures minimum mental stress for all former athletes.

Healthy Choices for Parents

A critical healthy choice for parents is guiding their children into a healthy lifestyle. There is a qualification required for this, however. You cannot give what you do not have. Parents need to first achieve a healthy lifestyle and then encourage their children to do the same. You cannot eat three scoops of fatty ice scream, frequently, for desserts and ask your children to eat fresh fruits and nuts for dessert.

Some children and young adults now eat different foods from their parents. In situations where these young people have researched or studied and found healthy fresh foods that they like, it is wonderful. There are situations, unfortunately, where these young people go by taste and what is popular with their friends and eat unhealthy foods. Some parents agree with these young people and accept the notion that the younger generation does not like healthy foods. Accepting this concept will boost the eating of unhealthy foods that may rapidly lead to the development of unhealthy weight with associated diseases such as diabetes mellitus and hypertension. This needs to be stopped before it grows into an epidemic.

It is intriguing to see some parents at groceries shopping with their children. Some of the children want to buy all kinds of unhealthy food items. Some parents refuse these items. I even saw a child who was about five years old present his case to the mom as to why the unhealthy food he wanted should be purchased. It was truly an interesting sight. Fortunately the mother stood her grounds and said no.

A healthy lifestyle is a gift parents can give to their children that can be passed down to future generations. It is one of those important gifts that keep on giving. The power of positive example can make a major difference in the health of families and ultimately the health of a nation.

Healthy Choices to Reduce Daily Injury Risk

Some basic precautions help to decrease injuries daily. These important precautions include:

- Bending your knees before lifting heavy objects
- Taking breaks if you have to type for several hours daily
- Holding onto rails while climbing stairs
- If you are sitting down for a long time, sit on chairs that support your back.

Social Habits Healthy Choices

Some social habits affect health. They can affect health positively or negatively. A social habit that affects health positively is dancing. Some dance moves count as exercise and have health benefits while some music have calming effects and reduce stress. Social habits that affect health adversely include alcohol consumption and smoking cigarettes.

The greatest problem with alcohol is control. Some people are social drinkers who drink limited alcohol at social events while others indulge in alcohol or binge on alcohol resulting in intoxication. No matter the intention, alcohol addiction starts with one glass of alcohol. Social drinkers increase alcohol consumption when their stress increases. Intoxication with alcohol results in serious consequences that range from impaired functioning to fatal accidents. Health adverse consequences of alcohol range from problems with medications to liver diseases such as liver cirrhosis. Some people seek to obtain health benefits from wine. The health benefits from wine can be obtained by drinking deep colored 100% grape juices such as red grape juice. It can also be obtained from eating deep red and purple grapes as well as other deep colored grapes. When intoxication from alcohol occurs, it can derail even the brightest of persons. No wonder in the Bible Book of Proverbs sometimes called the Book of Wisdom, it is written: "Wine is a mocker, intoxicating drink arouses brawling, and whoever is led astray by it is not wise." "Who has woe? Who has sorrow? Who has contentions? Who has complaints? Who has wounds without cause? Who has redness of eyes? Those who linger long at the wine: Those who go in search of mixed wine." (NKJB, Proverbs 20: 1; 23: 29-30)

Avoidance of alcohol and its adverse consequences is worthwhile. In so doing family crisis caused by alcohol consumption can be avoided. Fatalities due to drunk driving annually can be avoided as well. I know some people who quit drinking alcohol after finding themselves in devastating circumstances that resulted from being under the influence of alcohol.

Smoking cigarettes is extremely damaging to the body. It is a simple action that causes complex problems. Every effort should be made toward smoking cessation. Smoking adversely affects some medications. I tell patients while counseling them on medications that smoking while taking oral contraceptives, for instance, increases the chance of having a stroke. Smoking increases the chance of having blood clots and lung cancer. Air purifiers do not decrease the damaging effects of second hand smoke. Quitting smoking is the most profitable health decision that any smoker can make.

Action Summary # 13

Adhere to healthy choices and actions. Healthy choices and actions enhance overall health. A healthy lifestyle allows you to look good on the inside and on the outside. It promotes optimal function for your body and you will enjoy healthy skin and better vision. Your mood and immune system will be boosted. You will have good energy and a healthy mind. You will have reduced stress and you can sleep better at night. Avoid actions with the risk of injury.

The healthy lifestyle discussed, if followed, will also help to prevent the need for obesity surgery. This will in turn help to prevent possible morbidity and mortality associated with the surgery.

Seniors should avoid sedentary lifestyles. They should keep their minds and bodies active. They should also take medications safely by using pill organizers for multiple medications.

An athlete that focuses only on athletics is doing himself or herself a disfavor. Preparing for the next level in their lives after athletes, whenever that comes, cannot be overemphasized. Proper planning and adequate preparation ensures minimum mental stress for all former athletes following completion of athletic careers; whether the career ends in middle school or at the professional level.

Parents should strive to be examples of champions of a healthy lifestyle to their children. Healthy lifestyle by families will lead to healthier families and a healthier nation.

Avoid alcohol and its adverse consequences that include liver cirrhosis and some cancers. Smoking damages the body in numerous ways. Plan to quit if you smoke to improve your health and avoid certain cancers that are enhanced by smoking.

Chapter Fourteen

Seven Days Detoxification

Having seen the various ways that you can achieve a healthy lifestyle, you may want to take a break from your regular routine and try something new. It is one way to give your health a boost. It will impact your life positively and allow you to enjoy predictable beneficial results. This is, in a way, a chance to exclude all toxic foods and renew and rejuvenate your body with natural healthy foods.

Take a Challenge: Seven Days a Vegetarian Detoxification

Take a big step forward and go from your situation right now to a seven day challenge. During the seven days eat only fresh fruits, fresh vegetables, and a serving of nuts such as almonds or walnuts daily. You will obtain your daily vitamins in the best way recommended, by so doing. Also drink plenty of pure water as your beverage. Do some of the exercises we discussed earlier. Check your weight on the first day of the challenge. At the end of the seven days check your weight, energy level, and your overall health. Like Daniel, you will exceed your peers in energy and healthy look. You will also exceed them in a general feeling of wellbeing. You can then use the proven result as a motivation to make a healthy lifestyle your lifetime choice.

Seven Days a Vegetarian Detoxification

Detoxification involves the removal of toxic substances from the body. Various toxic substances in the body damage the cells of the body and can lead to the development of cancers. Toxic substances in the body that can damage cells include free radicals discussed earlier. Eating mostly raw and fresh fruits, vegetables, and nuts for one week decreases the chance of eating toxic foods, (as much as possible choose organic fruits and vegetables where recommended). Organic fruits and vegetables are free from toxins from pesticides. If you cannot afford organic fruits and vegetables wash the fruits and vegetables thoroughly. Do not just rinse them. Eating these will allow you the benefit of providing your body with needed antioxidants. Plasma levels of these substances will increase. Some of the vitamins for which I counsel patients are antioxidants found in brightly colored fruits and vegetables; including vitamin C, vitamin E and vitamin A. The pigment in these colors helps protect against certain diseases.

Macula is the center of the retina. Macular degeneration results from the additive effects of the damages that have been caused to the macula. It happens over time. It does not produce pain. Increase in macular degeneration decreases vision capabilities. When people have macular degeneration, there will be a blurred spot in the center of the image that they observe. Free radicals from different sources damage the eye. These sources include infection and sunlight. Sources of free radicals can also be pollution present in the air which includes cigarette smoke and other pollutants. The pigments from plants and vegetables (zeaxanthin and lutein) protect the eyes from the free radicals.

The eye lens is made up of a disc-like patch of proteins. This disc of proteins focuses light on the retina of the eye and as such affects vision. Retina is sensitive to light. Cataract is a clouding that occurs in the lens of the eye. When people get older they have an increased chance of developing cataract. When people have cataract, the image that they observe will be blurred and lack full detail due to the clouding of the lens of the eye. Zeaxanthin and lutein can help to protect the eye against cataract. These two pigments that are responsible for the deep colors of fruits and vegetables ensure the protection of your eyes. So the seven-day challenge will also boost the removal of toxic substances that can damage your eyes.

The fruits and vegetables that are sources of zeaxanthin and lutein include:

- Dark green spinach
- Dark green Romaine lettuce
- Collard greens
- Broccolis
- Grapes
- Kiwifruits
- Corns

Part of the benefits of the detoxification will be decreased constipation and the regulation of your digestive system and bowel movement. This will prevent the accumulation of toxins in the body from infrequent bowel movement. Improved satiation, decreased weight, as well as lower blood glucose will be part of the benefits during this period.

Water

Water is a very beneficial beverage. It makes up 65 to 70 % of your body weight. Water performs a lot of functions in the body which include the following:

(1) It helps to prevent constipation
(2) It makes available the moist environment needed by your eyes
(3) It provides moist environment for your ears
(4) It provides moist environment for your nose
(5) It provides moist environment for your throat
(6) It helps to transport nutrients and oxygen to various cells
(7) It helps to regulate the body temperature
(8) It helps to dissolve nutrients so that they can be available to the body
(9) It enhances the lubrication of your joint
(10)   It helps to provide moist environment for the tissues

Your sole beverage being water during this period will be profitable. The aches and pain that can occur in certain areas of the body due to inadequate water intake will be prevented. Dehydration will be prevented also. It is very easy for people to imagine big and scary medical problem sometimes, when the symptoms that they feel are simply due to poor hydration or dehydration.

Poor hydration or dehydration can result in the following:

- Constipation and cramping
- Leg cramp
- Headache
- Light headedness

When you are drinking enough water you will have colorless (clear) to very mild yellow urine. Deep yellow urine indicates that you are not drinking enough water or that you could be dehydrated.

Water and Detoxification

Water will flush toxins out of your body's vital organs which will decrease the burden on liver and kidneys. You could decrease your chance of developing bladder diseases through the intake of generous amount of water as well. Unfortunately, a lot of people live in a partially dehydrated state. The body shows certain symptoms when it is poorly hydrated. Pain and cramps due to inadequate hydration of the body are treated with over-the-counter medications by some people, instead of taking adequate fluid. Adequate hydration is also beneficial for the eyes. When the eyes are adequately hydrated and tear production is not hindered, the body benefits. This is superior to buying over-the-counter medication for dry eyes. The body can get rid of certain toxins through the tears. Adequate hydration boosts toxin removal from the body in various ways. As a result, during the seven days of detoxification your organs and tissues will function better and your health will be improved.

Exercise and Detoxification

We already know that exercise is a critical component of a healthy lifestyle. The benefits that exercise offer include detoxification of the body. As you exercise during the seven days include exercises that will make you sweat. When your exercises make you sweat, some of the toxins will be eliminated from your body through your skin along with the sweat.

Seven Days a Vegetarian Detoxification Reality

Once in a while I eat just fruits, vegetables, and nuts and drink water and 100 % juices just for one day. When I took the seven days vegetarian detoxifications challenge, eating only fruits, vegetables, and nuts and drinking water, I saw the difference that it can make. I ate six almonds after breakfast, six with lunch, and twelve at dinner. I made sure I was not hungry throughout the day. If I needed a snack, I had high fiber fresh foods such as carrots, celery, apples, and berries. I did the "excuse buster" exercise also most of the days. I exercised six out of the seven days for 30 to 45 minutes. I usually have a lot of energy. My energy increased even more than usual with the challenge. I felt lighter. I had even better gastrointestinal regulation benefit. It gave my wellbeing a boost. I lost two and one-half pounds during that week. I recommend this challenge to everyone. There is an excitement that comes with being up to a challenge. The first and second day may be more challenging but after that it will come naturally. Specific results may vary for each person but enhanced health will be true for everyone.

Recommendations for Fruits and Vegetables Availability

It is important and profitable to make fruits and vegetables more available especially to people who have financial difficulty. Some communities and organizations can donate their time or money to support growing vegetable gardens and some fruits. The produce from such gardens can be donated to those who need it the most. This will allow more people access to fruits and vegetables. The government can supports such endeavors by recognizing and supporting people who strive to make a difference in various communities in this way. Increasing the number of people who eat fruits and vegetables will help decrease the number of people with various diseases. This will in turn decrease the annual healthcare cost. Productivity will increase as well. Additionally, loss of time from work due to ill health will decrease.

Recommendations for Motivating People to Eat Healthier

Motivating people to eat healthier is a situation where everybody wins. If people eat healthier foods and adhere to healthy choices, they will be more productive in all their endeavors. They will lose less time and money to ill health. Some cereals list health benefits of eating them. People will feel really good and motivated if more of the fruits and vegetables, that are recommended, list their health benefits in addition to their contents. People will eat better if they know, for instance, the foods that enhance vision, digestive health, and heart health. The listing of calories and various nutrients that are contained in foods has been very beneficial to people. Addition of health benefits will motivate both sellers and buyers of foods to support healthy eating awareness.

Action Summary # 14

Take the seven days a vegetarian challenge. Eat only fresh fruits, vegetables, and nuts. Boost your health with various benefits from these foods. Take water as your beverage and obtain the detoxification of your body. Obtain relief from certain nagging pain with adequate hydration. Add exercise to further the detoxification of your body. The community can help to grow fruits and vegetable gardens that can be used to supply these foods to needy people.

Ending Comments

When all is said and done, one truth stands out. Effort made toward good health gets lavishly rewarded. It allows you to be healthy inside and look good outside. Healthy lifestyle dramatically and predictably reduces tissue and organ damage. Some terminal diseases can be avoided in the process of adhering to a healthy lifestyle. Aging process is slowed down as swell. The chance of living longer is increased.

One of the most important benefits of a healthy lifestyle is the ability to live an energetic life. It allows people to be more available for work and more productive at work. It greatly reduces the time that is spent resolving medical problems. It reduces healthcare related expenses as well.

Preventing diseases is more profitable than making frantic efforts toward treatment and cure. If health is maintained the right way in the beginning, the need for complicated treatments and procedures will decrease greatly. Healthy living will increase your peace of mind and reduce your stress level. It will make you more available for the things that you love and enjoy.

References:

(1) Dietary Supplement Fact Sheet: Vitamin A and
Carotenoids;
Http://ods.od.nih.gov/factsheets/VitaminA-
HealthProfessional   (Viewed 10/27/11)

(2) Dietary Supplement Fact Sheet: Folate;
Http://ods.od.nih.gov/factsheets/folate (Viewed 10/29/11)

(3) Dietary Supplement Fact Sheet: Vitamin B12;
Http://ods.od.nih.gov/factsheets/VitaminB12-QuickFacts/
(Viewed 10/29/11)

(4) Dietary Supplement Fact Sheet: Vitamin C;
Http://ods.od.nih.gov/factsheets/VitaminC-QuickFacts
(Viewed 11/5/11)

(5) Dietary Supplement Fact Sheet: Vitamin C;
Http://ods.od.nih.gov/factsheets/VitaminC-
HealthProfessional (Viewed 11/5/11)

(6) Dietary Supplement Fact Sheet: Vitamin D;
Http://ods.od.nih.gov/factsheets/VitaminD-QuickFacts
(Viewed 11/5/11)

(7) Dietary Supplement Fact Sheet: Vitamin D;
Http://ods.od.nih.gov/factsheets/VitaminD-
HealthProfessional (Viewed 11/5/11)

(8) Dietary Supplement Fact Sheet: Vitamin E;
Http://ods.od.nih.gov/factsheets/VitaminE-QuickFacts
(Viewed 11/5/11)

(9) Dietary Supplement Fact Sheet: Vitamin E; Http://ods.od.nih.gov/factsheets/VitaminE-HealthProfessional (Viewed 10/29/11)

(10)   Dietary Supplement Fact Sheet: Calcium; Http://ods.od.nih.gov/factsheets/Calcium-QuickFacts (Viewed 11/5/11)

(11)   Dietary Supplement Fact Sheet: Iron; Http://ods.od.nih.gov/factsheets/iron (Viewed 10/29/11)

(12)   Dietary Supplement Fact Sheet: Iodine; Http://ods.od.nih.gov/factsheets/Iodine-QuickFacts (Viewed 11/17/11)

(13)   Dietary Supplement Fact Sheet: Magnesium; Http://ods.od.nih.gov/factsheets/Magnesium-HealthProfessional

(14)   Dietary Supplement Fact Sheet: Zinc; Http://ods.od.nih.gov/factsheets/Zinc-QuickFacts (Viewed 11/18/11)

(15)   Dietary Supplement Fact Sheet: Zinc; Http://ods.od.nih.gov/factsheets/Zinc-HealthProfessional#en40 (Viewed 11/18/11)

These references are used with permission from the Office of Dietary Supplements of the National Institute of Health.

Please Note:

This book is not intended to serve as a diagnostic tool or for self treatment of any medical condition. If you are sick, promptly consult your physician. If you have a dental problem promptly consult your dentist. The information in this book is believed to be genuine and of premium quality, however, the author and publisher assume no liability for the use and misuse of the information provided in this book by the author. The information provided in this book should not be used as a substitute for proper medical attention.

Index